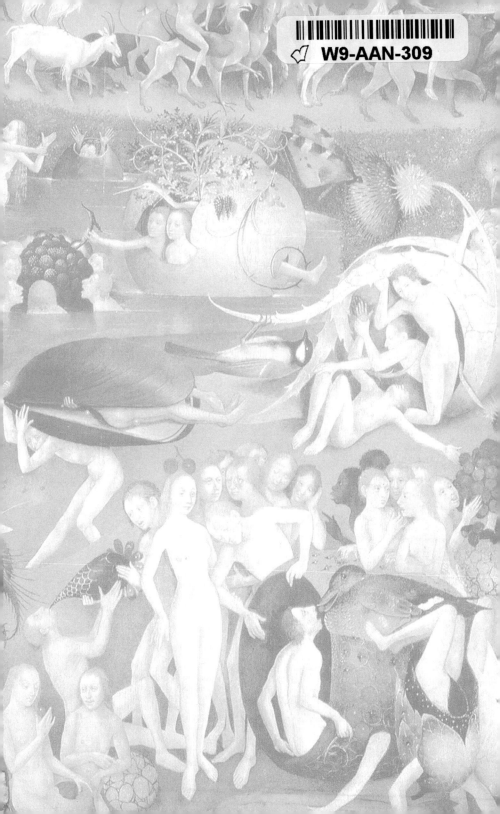

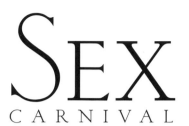

SEX
CARNIVAL

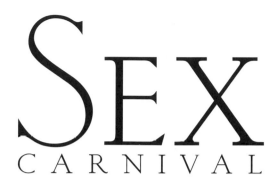

SEX
CARNIVAL

BILL BROWNSTEIN

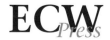

ECW *Press*

The publication of *Sex Carnival* has been generously supported by the Canada Council, the Ontario Arts Council, and the Government of Canada through the Book Publishing Industry Development Program.

CANADIAN CATALOGUING IN PUBLICATION DATA

Brownstein, Bill
Sex carnival
ISBN 1-55022-415-8
1. Sex-oriented business. 2. Pornography. I. Title.
HQ471.B768 2000   363.4'7   C00-931708-2

Cover image courtesy of The Prado Museum, Madrid.
Author photo by Barry Harris.
Cover and interior design by Guylaine Régimbald – SOLO DESIGN.
Typesetting by Yolande Martel.
This book is set in Dante and Sackers Light.

Printed by AGMV l'Imprimeur, Cap-Saint-Ignace, Quebec.

Distributed in Canada by General Distribution Services,
325 Humber College Boulevard, Etobicoke, Ontario M9W 7C3.

Distributed in the United States by LPC Group,
1436 West Randolph Street, Chicago, IL 60607, U.S.A.

Distributed in Europe by Turnaround Publisher Services, Unit 3,
Olympia Trading Estate, Coburg Road, Wood Green, London, N2Z 6T2.

Distributed in Australia and New Zealand by Wakefield Press,
17 Rundle Street (Box 2266), Kent Town, South Australia 5071.

Published by ECW PRESS
Suite 200
2120 Queen Street East
Toronto, Ontario M4E 1E2.

ecwpress.com

PRINTED AND BOUND IN CANADA

Contents

INTRODUCTION 11

LAS VEGAS
GETTIN' IT ON IN BABYLON 15

LOS ANGELES
DRIVIN' THE BULLS ON RODEO 39

NEW YORK
BITE ME! THE BIG APPLE 67

AMSTERDAM
BIKES, DIKES, AND BANANAS? 87

PARIS
MOULIN ROUGED 111

MONTREAL
TWO TONGUES ARE BETTER 125

CANADA
DON'T YA JUST LOVE
THIS FROZEN TUNDRA? 177

EPILOGUE 195

INTRODUCTION

"Explore," he urged over much saki and sushi.

"Like Magellan?" I replied. "Sorry. I don't do well where there are serpents or insects bigger than golf balls. In fact, I tend to limit my outdoor forays to golf courses, and I rarely traipse into the rough. Truth be told, I hail from folks who only explored out of necessity — mostly when they were being pursued through the steppes of Russia by saber-wielding Cossacks."

"Are you finished yet?" asked this most patient fellow, a publisher as it turned out.

The sort of exploration I'd described wasn't what he had in mind. He'd been intrigued by several newspaper columns I had written on the sex industry and some of the quirky people who populate it.

"I want you to explore the world of sex," he explained. "Go where your head and/or heart take you. And have fun. Are you ready to explore further?"

"Yeah, baby!" Amazing what sort of profound words leap into your larynx at moments like these. "And are you paying for this exploration?"

"To a point," he said, before spilling out the exact sum he was willing to invest.

"Well, there goes Bangkok," I responded. "But I'll have

plenty of time to explore North America and even a snippet of Europe. Right?"

"Not exactly," he shot back. "I need a finished book in six months."

"But, but . . ." I protested.

"Do you have much vacation time owing you?" he asked.

"Not exactly," I said. "It's the beginning of the year."

"So, do you like working weekends?" he asked.

"Not exactly," I said.

"So, I guess we have a deal," he said.

"We do?" I said.

And the moral of the story is: Never negotiate with a sage publisher over too much saki and sushi.

The sage publisher took his leave and I sat there in a stew.

"Are you okay?" an earnest busboy inquired.

"I'm not sure," I replied. "I've just undertaken to write a book about sex."

"Woo-hoo!" the busboy boomed in a voice that could raise the dead, even Magellan. "So," he asked, composing himself a little, "what do you know about the origins of sex? Where did it all begin?"

"I believe it was under a big old apple tree when some dude called Adam started canoodling with some babe called Eve," I muttered. "Now there are chat rooms on the Internet where hundreds of millions go to act out their fantasies. The lines have become blurred."

"That's it?" The busboy seemed incredulous.

"No," I said softly. "I don't believe that sex and saki mix. My lines have become blurred, too. My head hurts. Could you please call me a taxi?"

"You're going to need more than a taxi, my friend," retorted the busboy, suddenly concerned. He then invoked the very words that Eve is alleged to have uttered unto Adam some years back: "I don't think you have any idea what you've gotten yourself into."

Truer words were never spake, as Adam is alleged to have uttered unto Eve.

I English pretty bad. But I French pretty good.

— Exotic dancer April Showers, or possibly May Flowers

Chapter 1

GETTIN' IT ON IN BABYLON

The applause is near deafening as crowd favorite Tristan Taormino makes her way through a sea of admirers to the podium. She's picking up her award. "Oh, my God! This is so wonderful," she gushes, struggling to hold back tears and catch her breath. "Buttman, you gave me a chance when no one else would. The next thing I knew I was the subject of a ten-person anal gang-bang, and now this . . . I just want to thank my mom and dad . . ."

Damn, I missed the Céline Dion nuptials at Caesar's Palace, so I'll have to cover the porno Oscars at The Venetian instead. They say that sometimes you choose the job and sometimes the job chooses you. Okay, maybe it was me who said that. Whatever — that's my story and I'm sticking to it.

And so my odyssey into the wide world of sex begins with a sort of bang, because I can't get to the Palace on time to catch pop diva Céline Dion and her Svengali manager-husband, René Angelil, renew their marriage vows, in an event that can best be described as the Arabian Nights with a side order of falafel. The Caesar's Palace ballroom had been converted into a cluster of Berber tents. Adding to the ambiance of this $1.5 million wedding circus were several camels and jugglers and belly dancers. Clearly, pornography is relative. To many on this planet, an indulgent wedding circus with dromedaries and jugglers is more perverse than anything coming out of the adult-video biz — including a ten-person anal gang-bang.

Incidentally, Tristan Taormino's acceptance speech is prompted by her receiving top honors in the Best Anal-Themed Tape category at Vegas's annual Adult Video News (AVN) awards show. In a land where nothing succeeds like excess, there is likely little that is more excessive than the AVNs. Yet, like the porno biz itself, even the AVNs have become more mainstream. Heck, these days they even have a prize for Best Non-Sex Performance. The other categories and the stage names of the nominees might give one pause, but the ceremonies are pretty much standard issue — the same as any other awards orgy. Why else the stilt-walkers and tasteful Dixieland band at the entrance to the mammoth Venetian ballroom? Truly, this gala could pass for the Oscars or the Grammys. The vast majority of the 3,200 people in attendance are genteel, well-heeled, resplendent in their formal evening attire, and more intent on picking up shrimp at the buffet table than porno stars at the bar. Even *Screw* magazine's Al Goldstein and the infamous Joey Buttafuoco blend.

The emcee for the evening, adult star Julie Ashton, does her best to bring dignity to the proceedings. Which is not always an easy thing, particularly when Alisha Klass, last year's winner of the Best New Starlet award, comes to the stage and runs off at the mouth with a litany of legalese, illuminating the intricacies of binding contracts. But the only thing the audience notices is Klass's short gown, which has become unbound enough to reveal that she's wearing no undergarments.

Klass's ramblings aside, the level of humor here is certainly higher than the stale innuendo usually dished out at the Academy Awards, no doubt due to the fact that this show isn't being broadcast live on network T.V. "I thank you from the heart of my bottom," blurts Brit director Ben Dover after copping the AVN statuette for Best Gonzo Video — whatever that might be. "Why am I giving an award for best comedy?" barks comedy's pit bull, Bobby Slayton, a perennial AVN presenter. "Two things that don't really go together are the Three Stooges and sex. Trust me." Slayton continues: "Seriously, though, you have all accepted me as part of your family. And I want to be part of your family. Then we could all do Thanksgiving together and I could be stuffing Ginger Lynn and the gay guys could be stuffing the turkey. But no. I have to celebrate Thanksgiving with my wife. She doesn't understand this business. She doesn't like the girls. She says they're all idiots who just suck and fuck. I tell her: 'You're an idiot and you don't suck and fuck, so they're two steps ahead of you.'" Slayton concludes his rant on a relatively more philosophic note: "Does size matter? I think so. Personally, I don't like big pussies."

For the record, Slayton is more randy than any of the porno-biz presenters or recipients. Also for the record, *Double Feature* takes the prize for Best Comedy and cleans up in a host of other video categories as well, including Best Actor for Randy Spears and Best Actress for Serenity. In the film division — there is, apparently, some arcane distinction — *Seven Deadly Sins* is named the year's best, while the other big winners are Bonn (that's James Bonn) and Chloe, both for the feature *Chloe*. And honors for best acceptance speech — after Taormino's, that is — have to go to Zoe, cowinner of the Best Couples Sex Scene, Video. "I had no fuckin' clue I'd win this," she announces. "But I'd like to thank my costar, Van Damage, for letting me kick the shit out of him and then letting me fuck his brains out. He's a very generous actor. I hope he gets out of the hospital soon." A sentiment shared by nearly everyone in attendance.

There are many parallels between this glittering event and the various mainstream awards shows. Tedium, for one. But, unlike the Oscars, the AVNS always wrap on a high note. To demonstrate that there are no hard feelings, all the female

nominees leap onto the stage for some impromptu exotic dancing and occasional cuddling. And then one tries to imagine just
how much larger an audience the Oscars would draw if Whoopi
Goldberg and Jane Fonda committed a few naughty acts onstage.
Then again . . .

For the last sixteen years, the AVN awards have been held in
conjunction with the Adult Software Exhibits, which in turn
have been held in conjunction with the CES (Consumer Electronics Show) convention. Talk about strange bedfellows. The
Consumer Electronics Show mainly attracts distributors and
manufacturers from the decidedly unkinky world of high technology. Microsoft's billionaire brainiac, Bill Gates — someone
you never want to see having sex — has kicked off this year's
convention with a keynote address. Not to suggest that conventioneers aren't here to scope the latest in car stereos and
Internet-access devices, there is only one exhibit hall at the Sands
convention center, adjacent to The Venetian, and there's a
four-hour wait to enter. And they ain't lining up for automated
coffeemakers.

It is estimated that one hundred thousand people, many of
them digital dweebs, are eventually able to check out new
porno films like *Libido Loco* and *Screamin' for Seamen*, as well as
accessories like the smart Lavender Leather Ankle Cuffs, Vibrating Dong, or Anal Invader with Cock Cage. But the big buzz
among the gadget-grabbers is the Lorissa Love Doll, because,
as I hear one forthright young man succinctly put it, Lorissa
eliminates rejection and guarantees results for those with urges
and no time to waste in the mating process. And so what if
Lorissa is a piece of inert plastic that could pop under pressure?
"Check out the features," the fellow tells his buddy.

According to the specs, Lorissa is "a lifelike, ultrasoft, incredibly realistic doll with Futurotic vagina, anus, and mouth, made
from a new, three-dimensional, almost-seamless design providing added strength and a forming technique that creates a soft,
realistic-feeling skin. Real-life full mannequin head, supple,

customized-to-fit erotically noduled mouth, and a firm butt. Sensually scented. Removable multispeed vibrating bullet for extreme pleasure." And she never complains about insufficient foreplay, as our browser points out to his buddy. Yes, but does Lorissa do windows? Next, our funseekers patiently wait their turns to get autographs from, and pose with, such porno stars as Slutwoman, Buttman, Taylor Hayes, and Ron Jeremy, the chunky former schoolteacher whose fame is largely due to his ability to fellate himself. "Nice guy," the Lorissa-loving fellow tells his friend, "but, all the same, I wouldn't be shaking his hand if I were you — comprendo?"

Buoyed by record-breaking attendance figures, AVN publisher Paul Fishbein, who coordinates the awards gala as well as the Adult Software Exhibits, is now contemplating bolting from the CES and going solo. This will probably suit CES organizers just fine. Word is that its squeaky-clean exhibitors are becoming increasingly miffed at being overshadowed by the heavy traffic generated by porno stars in stilettos and little else. Frankly, they'd prefer that conventioneers gawk at Bill Gates, not Buttman. Whatever transpires, however, there is no question that the once-moribund porno biz is growing by leaps and bounds. More than ten billion dollars was spent on porno-related product in 1999 in the U.S. alone, up from $7.5 billion the year before. To put this in perspective, that is more than Americans spend on sporting events and live music combined, according to Frederick S. Lane III, author of *Obscene Profits: The Entrepreneurs of Pornography in the Cyber Age*. Oh, yeah, and chew on this bone: More than twelve thousand porno flicks were released in 1999 in the United States. And more than twenty-five percent of all video rentals in the U.S. came from the . . . mmm . . . back end of the shop.

Fishbein doesn't doubt the accuracy of these figures: "For the longest time, some people have been deluding themselves about the scope of the business. Believe me, it's not eight perverts out there renting all these films." Yet all of this pales in comparison with the latest hot source of adult product: the

Internet. Lane estimates that there are between thirty thousand and sixty thousand sex-oriented Web sites. And this doesn't even take into consideration the incalculable number of phone-sex lines and the chat rooms on the Net.

With the proliferation of specialty cable-T.V. outlets and the Internet the sky is the limit, according to Steven Hirsch, the owner of Vivid, the world's leading producer of adult films and videos. Vivid also owns two pay-per-view T.V. networks in the United States, The Hot Zone and The Hot Network, which reach an estimated audience of twenty-five million viewers. "We're properly positioned for the future," says the no-nonsense Hirsch, with no pun intended. Increasingly, more of those T.V. viewers, in addition to renters of adult videos, are women. Whereas women represented a minuscule portion of the market just a few years ago, they now fork over more than thirty percent of the cash spent on porno-biz products. And this is only the beginning. Listen up, ladies, gents, and gerbils, we have seen the future of porno, and it is that women will eventually rule. "And why not?" asks Vivid distributor Michelle Liss. "Today's films have plots and production values. Women don't have to be afraid of, or turned off by, them any longer. Besides, it's the new millennium. It's about time we had some fun, too."

At this fair, if not for all the sex wares and the ubiquitous porn stars on display, one could easily look around and get the wrong impression; these conventioneers could be, say, attending a livestock convention in Butte. Friendly, plainly dressed, fresh-scrubbed folks happily make the rounds. And nary a leer among them, even as they scope the spanking-new *Spankenstein* vid or the www.bondage.org Web site. The players in this biz also defy stereotype. Gold chains and greased-back hair are not what greet you here. A scene out of *Boogie Nights*, this ain't. Hirsch could easily pass for an accountant. His team of young execs looks like it was recruited from the Harvard Business School. "Make no mistake, this is a business like any other," Hirsch says. "We work hard. We're not breaking any laws. All we're doing is providing adult entertainment for an audience that wants to see it."

Put some clothes on her, and Teah, at a adjoining booth, could pass for a Classics prof at some Ivy League college. But Teah is more nimble than your average academic. Star of the flick *Asianatrix*, she is as adept with a bullwhip as she is with a checkbook, which explains why she has become a contract star with Typhoon Pictures. Like Hollywood luminaries of an earlier era, today's porn stars are contractually bound to their studios. But, unlike their Hollywood counterparts, few porn stars complain about the system. "I've worked both sides of the fence, and I honestly have to say the porn people are more genuine than the Hollywood types," says Teah, who has a degree in acting (fully clothed) from a reputable university. Clearly talented, she is able to converse about method acting while signing a publicity still — which depicts her fondling her breast with one hand and holding a delicate Asian parasol with the other.

Over at the next booth, xxxena, the impossibly well-endowed Empire contract star, attired in a tartan schoolgirl tunic, is not complaining either. Her physique can best be described as gravity defying, and she's intent on describing her boudoir skills. "I have lots of attributes, but I guess my best is deep throat," tosses out the star of *Insane in the Brain*. "I still can't believe that I get paid to do what I love most in life, which is to suck and fuck and lick . . . and the more, the merrier." A visitor to xxxena's stall asks if this is art. Without missing a beat, xxxena counters: "Only if you want it to be."

On the subject of art, many of the conventioneers and exhibitors are now repairing to Venice for lunch. Venice at the adjacent Venetian, that is. Here, the skies are permanently blue, the canals flow serenely, and gondoliers croon "O Sole Mio." Yup, this is Renaissance Venice in all its splendor — the art, the architecture, the arched bridges, the teeming piazzas, and the majestic stone walkways. All has been painstakingly and faithfully re-created within the walls of a vast hotel. Even Buttman and his entourage of big-haired babes are in awe.

And what's not to love? The canal water is crystal clear. There is no summertime Venetian stench, no gondola gridlock. And, of course, it never rains in this paradise. Visitors can sit, by day or by night, and lap up life at one of the cafés that line the piazza. Over lattes at one such establishment, Rick and Sue from Iowa — and not from the sex trade — discuss how this Venice is better than the real deal. Venice, Vegas-style, is cleaner and cheaper, they rhapsodize; the people are friendlier and English speaking, and the swell gondoliers never splash them.

At a nearby table, John Leslie reposes in a contented state. An icon in the porno biz, the soft-spoken, graying Leslie started out as a performer but has since moved behind the camera to direct some of the most art-laden erotica around, like the *Dirty Tricks* and *Voyeur* series. He's been called the Cecil B. DeMille of porno. His films have garnered more than one hundred AVNs over the years, and most of those were hard-earned in the days when the award categories were few and everyone was hungry for recognition. "Now everyone gets an award," he says over a martini. "It's become so watered down. I'm sure they'll soon give out a Best Anal Scene on a Thursday with Big Tits award. Really. Hell, they even nominated footage from one of my films for the Best Sex Scene award, and that scene never even happened."

One of Leslie's greatest pleasures is confounding people. "I am a very conventional man," he says. Many, even those not in the biz, call him a Renaissance Man. When not calling the shots on the set, he paints lush landscapes. He plays passionate harmonica in a blues band. He grows his own food. And he's been with the same woman for the last two decades. "The fun for me in sex films is putting the images together. But I have no illusions. I treat it like a canvas. But really, no matter what I do my work is being gobbled up by guys who only want it to whack off."

A couple approaches Leslie. She says he looks very familiar.

After they establish that Leslie isn't the real estate agent from Encino or the relative from Oakland, she turns beet red. "M-my Lord, you're him!" she stammers. "Who, dear?" her hubby inquires. "Oh, just someone I once saw in a movie," she mumbles. "Which movie, dear?" he asks. "I don't remember the name, hon-ey!" she shoots back. "Well, who else was in it, dear?" he asks, increasingly flustered. "Oh, never mind. Look, there's a singing gondolier — let's go for a ride," she says, tugging at his arm. "Should we ask him for his autograph before we go, dear?" he asks. "Would you just drop this right now, hon-ey?" she bellows.

The couple departs. Leslie has been practically oblivious to the entire exchange. But his significant other, Kathleen Nuzzo, is amused. "He gets this all the time," she explains. "People know him, but they don't know from where. And when they remember, they freak, usually because they're with someone who might not appreciate John's work." Nuzzo giggles. She is a nutritionist and a personal trainer by trade. She's also Leslie's CFO. Minds out of the gutter — that's chief financial officer of John Leslie's company, Curly Productions (don't ask).

Nuzzo met Leslie in 1980, at the peak of his career as a porno performer. "He was a huge star — well, you know what I mean," she says. "But it didn't bother me, because he could separate his work from his personal life. It's always been just a job for John. In the twenty years we've been together, he's never lied to me once. And I've never been jealous." Nuzzo has little reason to be; she is more radiant than most of the women Leslie has executed his boudoir acrobatics with. It also helps that she never watches his films (for that matter, neither does Leslie). Still, Nuzzo well understands Leslie's appeal — and again, it's not what you're thinking. "People love him because he brought a level of acting and integrity to his work," she says. "No one else in the business, except for Jamie Gillis, has ever come up to John's acting level. He could have been great in Hollywood. He could have so easily made the crossover. But by the time he was aware, he was already at the top of this business. He didn't feel like starting all over again." Nuzzo plays maracas in Leslie's blues band. "Audiences who hear his music would probably die if they knew what else he did for a living," she says. "Yet he's so much more at home playing blues on his mouth harp. That's where he's really at peace with himself."

These days, Leslie and Nuzzo attend the AVNs mainly to show solidarity. "The awards were more fun in the old days," she sighs. "Now you've got some girl going up on stage for her award, screaming: 'Fuck me up the ass and thanks for the honor!' What's that all about? That's why we now prefer to go to Budapest to make our movies and work with the talent there. It's a lot more classy." Before they split from the café, Leslie makes an odd observation: "With all the porno out there, is anybody having actual sex anymore? I really wonder."

Bobby Slayton, sitting one table over, pleads the Fifth Amendment on that one. He suggests that there's a downside to the fact that porno is becoming more accessible to the Middle American washed (unwashed?). "It takes all the fun out it. It's no longer a taboo. It's like tattoos. Every college douchebag has a tattoo now. They say it's a tribal thing. Right. Now everyone has accepted porno — everybody but my wife." Slayton is on a roll: "Some people think porno leads to violence against women. Wrong! It leads to a guy beating himself off. The guy then becomes too lazy to get off his ass to find the remote control for his television, let alone hurt anybody. What it really comes down to is this: porno leads to having a sandwich, which often leads to a nap."

While we are engrossed in conversation in this faux-Venetian café, an elderly gent in faux-Venetian period garb approaches Slayton. "I am Piccolini, and I am here to tell you that it's always sunny when you work in this Venice." Slayton is speechless. He doesn't know whether to pound the guy out or ask him for some of the Prozac he's obviously on. Buttman and Piccolini in the same room together. It's surreal. It's *The Truman Show*, is what it is. Then Slayton's eyes grow large, and it has nothing to do with Piccolini. A porn star he has admired from afar comes over to give him a peck on the cheek and inform him that she's no longer married. "So now would you consider me?" he asks meekly. "No," she sweetly retorts, "because you're still married, silly." As she retreats, Slayton shakes his head. "What's the world coming to? Even the porno chicks have principles and are monogamous these days. My luck."

Back down at the Adult Software Exhibits in the Sands convention center, I'm talking football with Bill Margold. He loves the Lions. I love the Giants. But since neither team has made it to the playoffs, Bill decides he can live with the Bills and the Colts, and so can I. Amazing. We're surrounded by the hottest porn stars and the most titillating new products the industry can muster, and, given our druthers, at this very moment, both of us would gladly beat a hasty retreat back to our hotel rooms to catch the Titans and the Bills on the tube.

Next, Bill and I shoot the breeze about nonporn films. He loved *The Green Mile*. I loathed it. I loved *Bowfinger*. He loathed it. Still, Bill and I have plenty in common. We're both called Bill. Also, we have both reviewed mainstream movies. But here the plot thickens. Margold started by writing reviews of mainstream features for such X-rated mags as *Cheri*, *Hustler*, and *Velvet*. I got my start by reviewing the oeuvres of Scorsese and Bergman and Fellini for the Canadian X-rated mag *Elite*. I was also paid to pen fake steamy letters to the editor for the same mag. Margold, however, has never had to stoop that low.

His penchant for football and mainstream movies notwithstanding, Bill Margold is a man on a mission at this convention. He's pretty much always on a mission. He's one of those individuals whom people like to refer to as a Renaissance man of porn (this biz seems to have more Renaissance men than the Renaissance ever did). But Margold prefers to call himself the grizzly bear of porn. Given his demeanor, however, I think teddy bear of porn is a more appropriate tag. And since this is my book, teddy bear it is. A large, hulking fellow, Margold has participated in virtually every aspect of the porno biz. He has written, performed, directed, and served as an agent. He has discovered the legendary Bunny Bleu, Serena, Seka, Kelly Nichols, Lee Caroll, and the inimitable Viper — the woman who broke Big Bill's heart, yet the only woman capable of proving that he had a heart to break in the first place. Margold's eyes grow misty at the mere mention of her name.

With Viper, Margold founded the X-Rated Critics Association. He dabbles in critiquing, as well — not only screen art, but also the industry itself. Cofounder of Fans of X-Rated Entertainment (FOXE) and a member of the board of directors of the Free Speech Organization (FSO), he has become the industry's unofficial watchdog. But if anyone has a problem, be it with a producer who won't pay or a performer who won't play it safe, Bill Margold is the man they seek out. He cares. Really. As overseer of Protecting Adult Welfare (PAW), he solves dilemmas the old-fashioned way. He gets mad. He also gets results. Because nobody wants to mess with the grizzly (I mean teddy bear) of porn, a man who has never met a committee he wouldn't join or an acronym he wouldn't attach his name to. Never at a loss for words, Margold sums himself up like this: "God created man. William Margold created himself."

Margold is in the midst of a conversation with attorney Paul Ramcharen, who happens to be the hubby of adult star Salena (*Hot Bods and Tailpipes*, *Shane's World*) Del Ray. "The work is tough," Ramcharen says. "Yeah, Salena just got a script with fifteen pages of dialogue. That's right — fifteen bloody pages. What's the world coming to when there are fifteen pages of fucking dialogue in a porno script?" Who the hell do these producers think they're dealing with — Meryl fucking Streep? Yeah, next thing you know producers will be forcing their performers to become method actors of the Lee Strasberg school and ditch the spontaneous primal groans. Sheesh. Bill Margold smiles. Briefly. "This is such a tough, soulless business," he murmurs. "It can, and will, eat most people alive. I counsel them to stay away from it altogether. You see, if you're not rebelling against something, you have no reason whatsoever to be in this line of work."

A doe-eyed young blonde comes to see Margold at his convention booth. She's been crying. Friends of friends have told her to get in touch with Bill. He's the only one who will help. To put it bluntly, she's been screwed in every imaginable way by an unsavory guy on the fringes of the biz. She needs money. And she needs a lift back to L.A. No questions asked, Margold makes the necessary arrangements — he'll give her a ride, a little cash. "There's no dollar sign in the word *cause*," he says. The girl's name is Angel. She poses in the buff for photos and does fetish nights. She has also been working as a production assistant on a few porno flicks. Margold tries, in his way, to comfort her. "Twenty-five years ago, this business was a family. Now it's a herd. Anybody can pick up a camera and make a movie. If someone left a camera in a gorilla cage for six months, he'd probably come up with a porno series called 'Banana Bonanza 1–6,'" he says, emitting a grizzly-sized laugh. "Point is, though, that in a business predicated on screwing, you're going to get fucked one day."

A small crowd has gathered to hear the teddy-bear-turned-preacher. "I love this business. I truly do. What I don't love is a lot of the people in it." Turning to Angel, he adds, "You want to make it. Well, you will simply have to sell me your soul, and then I'll make you famous. But understand one thing, dear: you have to be a sterile orphan in this racket. No family. No kids. Otherwise, one day your kid is going to come home from school carrying a magazine with a picture of you in the centerfold, lying down on a bed with a candle shoved up your ass. What are you going to tell your kid then, huh? That you were playing the part of a birthday cake? Right."

At this point, Angel looks like she's ready to crawl off to a convent. "Little does she realize that the entire four hours when I'm driving her back to L.A. she's going to have to listen to my tirades about the business as I try to talk her out of it," Margold says softly. Okay, Bill, let's cut to the chase. Is the porn industry any worse than the Hollywood film industry? "Oh, no," he replies in a nanosecond. "In Hollywood, you have to screw to get the part. In X-rated films, you only have to screw after you get the part. But at least you know what you're getting yourself in for."

Lo and behold, one of Margold's discoveries, the renowned Seka, makes her way through the crowd. She cuddles up to him. It's been fifteen years since Seka last performed her tricks with leaping lizards onscreen, and she doesn't miss the biz, not in the slightest. Semiretired and living in Chicago, Seka hasn't kept up with the latest developments. "I've heard [that the business] has rapidly evolved, but I wouldn't know. I never watch the films. In fact, I never even watched the films when I was making them. So why should I start now?" This much, however, she does know: "It's a business like any other." And this, too: "The X-rated world hasn't become more mainstream. The mainstream world has simply become more X-rated. Look around. Open your eyes. It's everywhere." To which Bill Margold adds his mantra: "Remember this: in a society that is drug-infested, violence-wracked, and polluted by chemical greed, no one has ever died of an overdose of pornography — unless they slammed their dicks in the VCR." Yeooouch! Gotcha.

Bill Margold hasn't spoken to Annabel Chong recently. For lack of a better term, Chong is a sexathalete. A marathoner. A real pioneer. In 1995, she broke what was then a world record by sleeping with 251 men in ten hours. Even though she's since been eclipsed, Chong is still dining out on this astonishing feat around the continent. She's also been busy promoting the flick that was spawned by her prowess: *Sex: The Annabel Chong Story*. No question, people are in awe. For example, upon learning of Chong's exploits, a concerned colleague of mine wished to know whether the athlete/actress smoked. If she did, he feared, her lungs would have also taken quite the licking. Well, Chong regretfully informed my buddy, she does smoke, but she didn't have a chance to light up between any of her 251 close encounters.

Chong, a native of Singapore whose real name is Grace Quek, would be the first to tell you that the title of her film is something of a misnomer, since it doesn't give us the definitive story of either sex or Chong. It does, however, tell us plenty about the rough-and-tumble world of porno. Directed by Torontonian Gough Lewis, *Sex* documents Chong's quest for horizontal fame, which she undertakes while studying fine arts at the University of Southern California and attempting to be a dutiful daughter. If this doesn't exactly compute in the minds of most, that's no surprise. Chong, who is now twenty-eight years old, is not your run-of-the-mill porno star. She is complex. She is unquestionably bright. And she is incredibly nonchalant about her feat: she was feeling bored; she wanted to explore her sexuality; and she didn't want to go through the whole pre-amble of foreplay to achieve her goal — otherwise she'd still be at it.

When it comes right down to it, *Sex*, while informative, is a fairly flaccid portrait of a young woman who seems depressed. Chong concurs: "These are the moments that Gough chose to put in the film, but they were just some of the moments we had in 130 hours of footage. Let's just say that the film is not really representative of me but that it does involve a lot of projection on the part of the director." We may jest about the hazards to Chong's health posed by smoking, but she wasn't in a joking mood after learning that not all of the men participating in the sex marathon had been tested for HIV, as the event's producer had promised they would be. "In my naivete, I believed everyone had been tested," says Chong. "The show has to go on, but at what cost?" Nor did one particular producer come through with the ten thousand dollars that Chong was supposed to be paid. "That really upset me, but rather than spend the time and energy pursuing the money, I went back to school to get my degree. And besides, I've made that money back in the business many times over."

After taking a brief hiatus from the porno biz, Chong is back, this time directing and producing, as well as starring in, her films. She can now laugh at the stories about how she and Gough Lewis were sexually involved during the making of *Sex*. The line is that Chong only had to sleep with one filmmaker, but other would-be stars have had to bed at least 251 to make it onto the marquee. "You know what they say in Hollywood: to get ahead, you have to give it," she cracks. "Sadly, it's all too true."

Reaction to Chong among feminist groups has run the gamut. Some have hailed her for being in control of her sexuality, while others claim that she has allowed herself to be victimized. She couldn't care less. "Feminism is such a nebulous term," she remarks. "What does it mean? Is it ecofeminism, radical feminism, lesbian feminism, or Marxist feminism? Regardless, they all hate each other and they all have their own dogma they try to impose. Anyway, men and women are equally oppressed when it comes down to it. To me, I'm a work in progress. I've made mistakes. But the important thing is that I've learned from my mistakes and I've moved on."

Chong is now directing a documentary followup to *Sex*. She says that it "won't be like *Die Hard 2* [an unfortunate example]. It will be another version of my life and address questions raised by [the first] film." One area Chong won't revisit in the sequel is excessive sex. She has no desire to enter another marathon. In fact, by the time I spoke to her, the record she'd established had already been broken three times — first by Jasmine St. Clair, then by Spontaneous Ecstacy, and finally by Houston, who managed to have sex with 620 men in six hours. "That's nothing," Chong says. "A woman called Montana plans to do two thousand men in honor of the new millennium. It's getting a little ridiculous. In a few years from now, we'll have the technology to break these records without men. We'll have just computers and a virtual gang-bang."

Annabel Chong meet Candy Apples. By a quirk of fate, they miss one another — which might be just as well — but I do catch up with Candy Apples at the CES convention in Vegas. She doesn't want to know from computers and virtual gang-bangs just yet. Not while she's still in a position — on her back — to set records. A buxom blonde who could pass for the girl next door — provided you live next door to Elly May of *Beverly Hillbillies* fame — twenty-six-year-old Candy Apples is the picture of innocence. Only a few tasteful tattoos on her torso detract from that impression. So, imagine my surprise when I learn that Candy Apples has made it into someone's annals (not likely those of Mr. Guinness) for having survived a 742-man gang-bang one day in Los Angeles during the final moments of the millennium. Hold me up. No, better still, hold her up. Apples is the fourth to break Annabel Chong's seemingly unbreakable record of 251. But times change, and so do appetites.

"I could have done a lot more, too," she says, smiling ever so sweetly. "But the blasted cops busted the show." They clearly had no appreciation for Candy's breathtaking endurance and athleticism. Candy Apples is still sore. But not from the marathon ordeal — rather from the indignity of having her freedom of expression violated. "We weren't hurting anyone," she insists. "All we really wanted to do was set a world record that would have been impossible to break." Evidently, someone has already set the record. We're guessing that it's the aforementioned Montana. "She claimed she did two thousand guys," says Apples, "but my spies say it was more like thirty-five guys coming back for more. Whatever. There's no way she did two thousand guys. No way." Candy Apples is sounding sour apples.

Not that she needs to mention this, but Candy Apples wants the world to know: "I really like sex. Really." Prior to becoming obsessed with quantity, Apples focused her energies on quality. Sort of. She spent seven years as a performer in the porno-film biz, accumulating more than five hundred credits. Like Annabel Chong, Candy Apples is mindful of the health risks involved in bedding 742 men. She, too, demanded that all of her marathon partners be screened in advance and that they wear condoms. And once the deed was done, Candy Apples took a two-month break from the business of competitive sex and went into "quarantine" at her home in Huntington Beach, California.

She didn't swear off sex completely, though. Her one exception was her hubby, Bill Apples (who has taken on his wife's professional last name — it's better for business). Bill and Candy Apples were married right after Candy's big gang-bang. In fact, Bill was the last poker at the proverbial plate for the bang. "I thought it was romantic," he now says. "Me too," coos Candy. Sometimes you choose the apples, and sometimes the apples choose you.

The Apples say they're contemplating kids to fill up their family barrel. And then the words of Bill Margold come back to haunt: What will they say to their kid when he comes home from school one day and confronts them about their past? But Bill Apples has other preoccupations right now. He has become Candy's manager, and he's mighty bullish about her prospects, particularly since her recent surgical enhancement. "I just got a boob job," says Candy, flashing her new apples . . . er . . . the results of the procedure. "We believe that will really help her," Bill adds. "Also, I've been watching what I eat," says Candy Apples. Mr. and Mrs. Apples both giggle at that remark.

"If I could offer one piece of advice?" Okay, go ahead Candy Apples. "I can't stress how important it is to look after yourself — and not just in my business but no matter what vocation you choose. After all, you only go around once in life." Yeah, except for those in the employ of Montana.

With all due respect for the work ethic of Annabel Chong and Candy Apples, some in the porn biz maintain that a jaded public needs new thrills, beyond the endurance records and beyond the contrivances presented in most adult videos. They want reality. They want to peek at couples caught in the act of smut. It comes as no shock, then, that the hottest new vids circulating around the Vegas trade show, indeed around North America, are *Lovers Caught on Tape* and its sequel, *More Lovers Caught on Tape*. These compilations of the titillating sexual escapades engaged in by people who are generally oblivious to the fact that they've been caught with their pants down — and then some — are made possible by the closed-circuit video camera.

So, sing along to the refrain that's being sung at trash counters everywhere these days: "They're going to put you in the movies / They're going to make a big star out of you / You'll play the part of a man who's really horny / And all you've got to do is . . . get yourself a great divorce attorney." With apologies to the Beatles for bastardizing one of Ringo's only known hits, the aforementioned scenario is no longer the stuff of fantasy. Not when it turns out that the Cecil B. DeMille of tomorrow is, as paranoiacs have always suspected, Big Brother. Of course, you may know this person better as the genial security guard stationed in your office or apartment building, the dude at the desk whose eyes are glued to that console of video monitors. And now you know why.

Not everyone is aware that their elevator or parking lot or laundry room is equipped with hidden video cameras. And sometimes, after unwinding over a few drinks, neighbors or coworkers can take leave of their senses and do the darndest things. *Lovers Caught on Tape* and *More Lovers Caught on Tape* are the X-rated versions of *America's Funniest Home Videos*. The footage is fairly explicit. Much foreplay, much fellatio, much shtupping, some same-sex (women, natch) frolicking, and little in the way of subtlety. Only some of the faces have been blurred to ward off lawsuits. In those sequences where the faces remain identifiable, the players have signed release forms, usually for serious wads of cash and almost always because they're doing the nasty with their principal mate.

Evidently, what excites consumers of these videos is that the actors aren't pros pretending to be aroused. Real people are in real heat here, and that's the turn-on, according to Bobby Logan and Eric Riddley, the earnest-looking young entrepreneurs who produced the *Lovers* videos and who are manning a booth at the Vegas trade show. Logan and Riddley purchase their material from detective agencies and private security firms throughout North America. Actually, the *Lovers Caught on Tape* series is a natural extension for the boys. Prior to dabbling in candid porno, they brokered footage for network caught-on-camera shows like *Busted on the Job* and *Shocking Behavior*. "Essentially, the *Lovers Caught on Tape* material was stuff that the detective agencies and security firms couldn't sell and that the networks wouldn't touch," Logan explains. "So we ended up with all this backshelf footage and decided to do something with it." Within weeks of the release of the two videos, sales had reached more than fifty thousand copies. There are plans for one more. "But then we're out of footage," sighs Logan. "I'd love to be able to capitalize on the craze. But the sad reality is there just won't be *Lovers Caught on Tape 18* to hit the market. Our customers will be really disappointed, too. They've really become hooked on this stuff."

Small wonder, says Ray Pope of vmc Entertainment, the adult-video company that owns the film's exclusive distribution rights in Canada. "It's the whole unpredictable aspect that fascinates people," he opines. "It's similar to the public's fascination with T.V. shows with actual car crashes and chases." What makes Pope particularly proud is that one *Lovers Caught on Tape* sequence dispels the myth that Canadians are about as exciting as frozen cowpies. Canadian flag-wavers were delighted to see revealing footage of a couple ignoring the onfield action at Toronto's SkyDome and getting into the physical-fitness spirit all on their own. "Now nobody will ever be able to say that Canadians don't really enjoy baseball," Pope says.

Logan and Riddley, along with Pope, insist that they have conformed to U.S. and Canadian government regulations requiring them to obtain written consent from the folks whose faces are clearly displayed in their flicks. "We tracked down all those people from the tapes," Logan explains. "What's left on tape is footage from the people who didn't tell us to go straight to hell." But then there are the bodies of those whose faces have been blurred. Their presence raises the sticky question of what happens when someone — say, a spouse — recognizes a body part of his or her significant other. Presumably, it is at this juncture that the lawyers move in for the kill. Yet Logan and Riddley's VidBidness Inc. hasn't been hit with a lawsuit to date.

Which gives rise to another question. Has this stuff been staged? Riddley bristles at the suggestion: "I'd venture to say that ninety percent of what we get is totally real. On the other hand, a lot of the other stuff I've seen screams fraud right from the get-go. But this business is a tough nut to crack. You have to have your contacts, and we work with a network of three thousand private detective agencies and security firms around the world."

If there is a lesson to be learned here, it's that we should all be aware that we're almost never alone. Video scrutiny is rampant. "In a perfect world, I wouldn't want someone secretly monitoring my every move," Pope says. "But, face it, these hidden cameras aren't set up to catch people having sex. They've been set up for security purposes. Point is, you have to keep your head up in the new millennium. I now know a lot better after having seen this tape." Well and good, but where does all this voyeurism end? Do we have to fear that hidden cameras are lurking in private bedrooms?

In a word: yes. Pope says his company has been offered videos featuring funky couplings in the bedroom, bathroom, locker room, and other locales we've previously assumed were private. "If it's been illegally obtained — which material taken from such places is — we pass," Pope states. Same, too, for Logan and Riddley. "We have legal issues with that," asserts Riddley. "Still, most of the stuff they say comes from these illegal spycams is staged. I've even had porno actresses come up to me and say they've been hired to perform in these so-called candid sequences." The guys do grant, however, that not even strict privacy laws have deterred some from marketing this sort of material on the Net or via mailorder. "They just figure they'll move much faster than the law," says Pope.

Still disturbed at the notion that trusted security guards might be privy to more than they let on, I do an informal survey of several downtown office and apartment buildings. When asked if they've ever witnessed any X-rated antics on hidden cameras, all of the security guards I poll say no. However, not one of them expresses any surprise that such material exists. As one so delicately puts it, "If you have the urge, you have the urge — and nothing, not even a camera, is going to stop you. Who thinks anymore?"

Those in the know, that is, those whose job it is to document deep cultural developments, have suggested that the public's fascination with videos that peep at the lives of ordinary people all began with a pair of allegedly extraordinary celebs: Pamela Anderson and former hubby Tommy Lee. *Pam and Tommy Lee: Stolen Honeymoon*, clearly not your standard Niagara Falls tryst, emerged in 1998, and it's still hot stuff at some of the Vegas trade-show outlets. With the release of this video, some say the sanctity and privacy of marriage went by the boards. Why Pam (definitely more of an actress than she's ever been given credit for) and Tommy (a heavy-metal musician and an acrobat who somehow managed both to film and perform in the video), would decide to share with the world some of their most intimate moments is a perplexing question. But the fact of the matter is that the couple had little choice.

Learning that Web geeks the world over were gawking at their purloined private property, which had been bootlegged and released on the Internet, Anderson and Lee went to court in an effort to halt all this activity. But they lost their bid to have the video banned. They then forged an agreement with a distributor that at least allowed them to profit from what they considered their best work in years. Well and good, but while the presskit that accompanies the video boasts of much explicitness, and while the cassette cover itself suggests an inordinate amount of kink, the video in the box I pick up is a bust. Perhaps the most interesting aspect of *Pam and Tommy Lee: Stolen Honeymoon* is that it comes in two flavors: sexually explicit and R-rated. I'm not sure which one I have. Whatever it is, it features very little revealing material. All I can now say for certain is that Tommy has tattoos and Pam can swim and moan simultaneously. Not exactly, well, thumbs-up stuff.

The video does contain an element of mystery, however. There's Pam, all right, naked and frolicking. But there's little hard evidence of Tommy. Let me rephrase that: there is plenty of hard evidence (Dirk Diggler, eat your heart out) but none that proves beyond the shadow of a doubt that the private part being examined by Pam belongs to her beloved husband. Tommy's story is that he couldn't very well get a shot of his head while filming the action at the southern reaches of his body. Fair enough, but some investigative journalists harbor doubts. Maybe the next time Tommy embarks on a honeymoon he ought to leave the home-video camera behind and consider consummating the marriage in an elevator. This would ensure that all of him gets into the frame and put to rest any rumors that he employs a lower-body double.

Having completed my rounds of the CES convention, in the process wearing out my eyes and feet, I return to Bill Margold's booth to bid him adieu. He senses, accurately, that I am somewhat disillusioned or bored or tired or all of the above. He suggests a quick visit to Los Angeles. For high in the Hollywood hills, there lives a somewhat reclusive fellow who figured it all out years ago. That is, the public's fascination with seeing the likes of Pamela Anderson and other shapely starlets buck naked. So he captured their essence in a magazine, and the only thing that separated us from them was a few staples. His name is Hugh, and he lives in a mansion with a lot of wildlife.

Chapter 2

DRIVIN' THE BULLS ON RODEO

Terry is a twenty-eight-year-old wooly monkey. If Terry could talk, my gosh, would this simian have tales to tell. Terry has spent pretty much her entire life in a preserve on the grounds of the Los Angeles Playboy Mansion in Holmby Hills. She has witnessed a procession of movie stars gettin' wet and makin' whoopee in the Grotto. Terry has been petted by almost as many Playmates as her owner, Hugh ("Please call me Hef") Hefner, the founder of *Playboy* and still a hipster after all these years.

This wooly monkey has also been there for the low points. The highly publicized murder of Playmate of the Year Dorothy Stratten in the early eighties. Hef's struggle to shake off the effects of the stroke he suffered in the mid-eighties. Terry was likely incredulous, too, when Hef tied the knot later in the decade with Playmate Kimberly Conrad and then sired two sons. And Terry must have watched in awe as Hef separated from Kimberly and became a swinger again in the late nineties, taking up with those cuddly twins, Sandy and Mandy Bentley, as well as Brande Roderick — whose combined ages at the beginning of the millennium still left them ten years younger than their shared beau. These days, Terry is doubtless scratching her head in wonder at the news that Hef has added two more twenty-something babes, Jessica and Amy, to his roster of admirers.

And right about now, Terry probably wishes Hef would share his Viagra with some of the other monkeys in the cage. Terry, you see, just might be the only critter at the Playboy Mansion who ain't gettin' any. Even the peacocks prowling the grounds are getting boinked with regularity. It's their mating season. This we know, because their feathers are fanned out and they're particularly gnarly. While it's best not to mess with the peacocks or, for that matter, with Terry the wooly monkey, only one human has ever been bitten by a simian of Hef's. No one knows whether the chomper was Terry, but the human on the receiving end was a lawyer and few tears were shed for him.

The Playboy Mansion is Disneyland for adventurous adults — at least those who are deemed worthy by Hef. On this six-acre spread, a bevy of Playmates coexist with exotic monkeys, birds, iguanas, and fish, as well as less exotic cats and dogs and (naturally) rabbits. It's a world away from the hustle-bustle of nearby Sunset Boulevard. There is a game house on the property equipped with Playboy pinball machines and a pool table and a functioning Wurlitzer and a playroom with — nudge, nudge, wink, wink — a mirror-ceilinged reclining area. A staff of seventy tends to the needs of Hef, his animals, and all their pals.

At the Playboy Mansion's gated entrance, a talking rock inquires as to the nature of your business. And if you pass the skill-testing question it poses, the talking rock will trigger the opening of the gates. After a short ride up the hill — Playmates at Play caution signs line the drive — you arrive at Hef's ornate English-style manor. Built in 1927 by some Brit-lovers, the mansion reflects the Tudor, Gothic, and fourteenth-century Scottish Perpendicular architectural styles. No doubt those original residents are spinning in their final resting places due to all that fornication taking place inside (and outside) the manor's hallowed walls. Then again, maybe those ghosts, too, are, just wishing they could join the party. And, make no mistake, every day's a party here because that's what the Playboy image demands — and, more to the point, that's what Hef, the unreconstructed party animal, wants. The party can take the form of an all-out Viagra Valentine's Day affair for which the stars come crawling out of the fourteenth-century Scottish Perpendicular woodwork or a serene screening of silent films for the members of Hef's weekend movie club.

On that note, it is with a particularly heavy heart I must report that on the day of my visit Jack Nicholson is not fondling Charlize Theron in the Grotto, James Caan is not chasing someone called Bambi across the manicured lawn, Leonardo DiCaprio is not sucking face with Courtney Love, the Foo Fighters, or Liam Neeson. And where is that old coot Tony Curtis when we really need him? Or even those bad-boy Baldwin brothers? Not even Kato bloody Kaelin, for goodness sakes. No one — and I checked thoroughly — but no one is copulating in the corridors of the Playboy Mansion on this spring day. Perhaps because it is unseasonably blustery. I guess I'll just have to console myself with a fleeting glimpse of Playmate of the Year Jodi Ann Paterson in the driveway — she's leaving the premises following a vigorous workout in the gym. Or a quick brush with the assistants to Bill Maher, who is broadcasting *Politically Incorrect* live from the Playboy Mansion this week.

Bill Farley, Hef's genial longtime PR man, tells me not to feel bad. During his first day on the job, Farley was buttonholed by a Playmate at a party. She took him to a private room, where she proceeded to show him a series of revealing photos of herself. Then she excused herself for a minute, promising to return anon. Farley waited and waited and fantasized about the skimpy attire the lady was slipping into just for him. But, damn, she never returned. And Farley swears that this is as close as he's ever come to experiencing an encounter of the intimate kind at the Playboy Mansion. Still, people are forever

assuming that he gets pampered by the Playmates. So as not to
disillusion them or undermine the image of the place, he tells
callers who ask what sort of frolicking he's up to at the moment that he's lying in a hot tub getting massaged by the most
voluptuous Playmate. Because a guy's got to dream, right? And
reality — well, no one wants to know about it.

Farley escorts me to the Playboy Mansion library, which is
filled with an inordinate number of film books and more than
four thousand feature-length flicks. Hef, it seems, loves the
movies almost as much as he loves the ladies. Farley ushers me
to a sturdy armchair and offers me a vintage bottle of Playboy
water. And then Hef shows up, exactly as billed, sporting black
pajamas and red smoking jacket and clutching a Diet Pepsi. He
seats himself delicately on an adjoining sofa. Even if he has had
a few surgical nips around the face, as goes the buzz, he looks
grand for seventy-four. The mind, too, is clearly in good working order. Some would love to believe that Hef has become
some senile fart like Colonel Sanders, wheeled around on a
gurney and manipulated like a puppet by his minions. But such
is not the case. Hef is feeling pretty good about himself and
about life in general these days. And why not? He's in vogue
again and he's lappin' it all up.

The man who headed the vanguard of the American sexual
revolution has been both deified and vilified since establishing
his empire back in 1953. That's when he published the first issue
of *Playboy*, which featured a fab calendar photo of Marilyn
Monroe. The magazine begat clubs and casinos and resorts,
which begat film, T.V., and video operations, which begat surfing and E-commerce on the Internet. But these days Hef leaves
the running of Chicago-based Playboy Enterprises to his daughter, Christie Hefner; he mostly concentrates on perpetuating
the Playboy philosophy and editing the magazine.

"I'm glad to have lived to see the shift in the winds," comments Hef. He considers his words carefully before uttering
them. He is decidedly understated, almost bashful in his
demeanor. "We had a conservative backlash in the eighties and

early nineties, which was a response to all the dramatic changes of the sixties and seventies. Now we're getting a whole new generation who haven't bought into the political correctness and the moral majority." Hef, who is rarely astonished, is astonished that some of the women who wanted to crucify him a few decades back are now crediting him as being a contributor to the women's liberation movement. Hef, who rarely raises his voice, raises his voice a tad: "That has been a revelation and the most satisfying part of all. That's a postfeminist phenomenon. The feminist movement got caught up in this puritan, antisexual agenda, which didn't make a lot of sense and, for a new generation, doesn't make a lot of sense. One of the things that happens with political movements is that [they] attempt to lose [their] sense of humor and humanity. That's what happened to a portion of the women's movement." Hef raises his voice a little more: "From the outset, I never said that only men should have a good time. The plan included women as well."

According to Hef, the centerfold makes as strong a political statement as the Playboy philosophy does. "What it says is that nice girls like sex, too, that it's a natural part of life." Indeed, some nice girls even like sex more than nice boys. Hef chortles. Not only is he pleased with the fact that women's attitudes towards *Playboy* have changed, but he's also delighted that the once-cursed Bunny emblem has lately been embraced as a sort of icon. Check out the stories in *Vogue, Cosmo, Harper's Bazaar,* and *Vanity Fair,* he implores. He speaks of one such piece, by an archfeminist, which tells the Playboy Club story favorably from a Bunny's point of view. "For so long their story had simply been held hostage by a political agenda that came from Gloria Steinem." Even invoking the name of that famed feminist [once a Bunny herself] makes him wince.

Want to get a real rise out of Hef? Say "exploitation." In reference to Hef making his daily bread off the breasts and butts of the buxom babes who fill the pages of his magazine. "The term 'exploitation' has become a catchphrase that's rather like

Orwellian newspeak. What does it mean? To understand that, you have to look at American history and see how that puritan element of our culture started. It's as American as apple pie." Hef eschews clichés, but this one is apt. Hef also knows a thing or two about puritanism. He comes from a puritan background. "You betcha," he beams. "That's why I know it. It was there in my home." The elder son of ultraconservative Glen and Grace Hefner, Hugh is also a direct descendent of such pedigreed Massachusetts Puritan patriarchs as William Bradford and John Winthrop.

Hef is well aware of what his enterprise has unleashed. While he isn't turned on by today's extreme porn, he also doesn't apologize for blazing a trail for it. "I think someone's going too far every day, but that's what you get with democracy. It's a dangerous concept — still, it's the best one. Of course, there should be some limitations, but to what's truly hurtful and not someone's political agenda. When the subject was sex, the laws didn't really have much to do with what we call 'moral' or what was good for the people. It had to do with religious values, the whole notion being that the only moral purpose of sex was procreation. Those values are still in place in terms of birth control and abortion around the world, and here we are on a small planet suffering from a population explosion." He concedes that times have changed dramatically since the dawn of *Playboy*. "Sure, we're more tolerant, but we still remain a puritan people in many respects. What's had the biggest impact on sex in the last century is technology. Inventions that arrived with electricity — like motion pictures, radio, T.V., and the Internet — have turned us into a global village and have demystified sex. Pandora's box is open."

Few have benefited more from these contemporary innovations than Hef himself. To many, he is still the living embodiment of fun — an image he just loves to project. At an age when many of his contemporaries are incontinent or in retirement homes, Hef is out there playing like a kid. People half his age envy him his harem. Hef reflects on this and then spouts a little H.L. Mencken: "A puritan is someone who believes that somewhere someone is having a very good time." He lets out a cackle. "I'm doing the best I can. Living well is the best revenge." But there's no time to waste gloating. Hef has a message: "All of what has happened in my life has not made me cynical, has not made me overly sophisticated or jaded. I am still very much the boy who dreamed the dreams and stayed connected to them. It's just been a grand and magical adventure. Sometimes people ask me if my life is as good as it seems from the outside and the honest answer is that it's better. I'm a romantic and an idealist. Sure, you get the bumps in the road — but I still wear my heart on my sleeve, because that's part of it, too."

Hef and his entourage have been working diligently of late to recapture the party spirit that prevailed at the Playboy Mansion in the early days. "This place has been referred to as a Shangri-La . . . It's a place of dreams and fantasies. But at the same time it's a place with very real rules. Women are safer here than most any place in L.A. People get out of line here and they're gone. That's real morality. I said a long time ago that I'm the most moral millionaire I've ever met. People say power corrupts. I think it's a test." Yes, but morality aside, it has to be a thrill to vault back into the limelight. Hef doesn't hold back. "It's been like having died and then come back." The way he sees it, he didn't fall out of public favor; he voluntarily abandoned the scene to experience wedded bliss with his second wife, Kimberly. (Hef was married for a short spell in the early fifties to his college sweetheart, Mildred Williams, mother of Christie and son David.) But bliss was not to be after almost nine years of marriage. "Then it was like Elvis reappeared at the supermarket. That was coupled with a whole new generation growing up and [getting] tired of the political correctness and repression of the eighties and early nineties."

So the party got kick-started again, and Hef was there to greet the new millennium with babes on both arms and other appendages. Of course, it didn't hurt that his ascent coincided with the ascent of Viagra. "Timing is everything in this business, too," he cracks. "I have a great interest in Viagra. My marriage ended in 1998 and I got my first prescription for Viagra on my birthday a few months later." Best damned birthday present he ever got, he'll tell you. "When you have five girlfriends, you need it. It's much more than Pfizer suggested it was, too. It's more than an impotence drug. It's the best legal recreational drug out there — for me. It takes away the gap between your expectations and your fantasies." Spoken like a man with a stake in Pfizer and five young women to satisfy. And yet, while he admits that sex remains the single most enjoyable part of his life, it must have a context — romance, for instance. As stated, Hef is an incurable romantic. That might not be the image others have of him. "People project a great deal of their own fantasies and prejudices onto my life. *Playboy* reflects a portion of the sexual phenomenon where we do have so many fantasies and guilt." Which is to say that Hef makes a distinction between sex and smut. "I'm aware of where the market has gone. I look at *Penthouse*, and I know they're hardcore now. I see the hardcore videos that are out there — some of them are part of my entertainment."

Hef views his somewhat sanitized notion of sex — and not religion — as the major civilizing force on this planet. "It brings couples together. It forms families. If there weren't two sexes on this planet, what a cold, lonely place it would be." That sort of talk makes Hef sound almost like a man of the cloth, yet this was the guy who was branded a pornographer in the fifties. The guy who had to go to court to fight for a second-class mail permit for his magazine. The guy who had to go to court to fight for liquor licenses for his clubs. The guy the authorities tried to prosecute for obscenity and target as a drug dealer. And yet today no one's granny is even going to raise her eyebrows at *Playboy* pictorials of wholesome college girls who pose topless and occasionally bottomless. Hef has raised, or lowered, the bar. "I was so high profile in certain quarters. Look, they also went after Al Goldstein and *Screw*, and Larry Flynt and *Hustler*," he says, and then he adds, with a laugh: "If you look at *Playboy* with the virtue of hindsight, after almost five decades, you will find that there's almost nothing in the magazine that anyone would seriously object to — unless they're coming from a very strange quarter. The magazine, from my perception, has never been a sex magazine. I attempted to put together a lifestyle magazine for young men and incorporate it with the primary thing that young men were interested in. So to leave out the opposite sex for me would seem bizarre. To simply produce a sex magazine would be, in my opinion, to do nothing. Everybody does that. But to incorporate it as part of the acceptable fabric of the human experience and to give it style and context — now that's something."

Ultimately, Hef sees himself as Mr. Decent. Which is why he bristles at the accusations that were leveled against him by Peter Bogdanovich in a book and on the talk-show circuit. Film director Bogdanovich is a former buddy of Hef's. He hung out at the Playboy Mansion a few decades back. He implied that the Playboy lifestyle was responsible for the death of Playmate Dorothy Stratten, in spite of the fact that she was killed by her manic and jealous husband, Paul Snider. Stratten was trying to end her marriage and settle down with Bogdanovich. A somber Hefner explains that the director's accusations were "an attempt to assuage Bogdanovich's own sense of guilt, to make sense of something that was inexplicable. Maybe on a more cynical level it was an attempt to gain approval from the anti-Playboy, anti-sexual feminists. He attempted to change the laws of obscenity in America — but unsuccessfully." All of this was compounded for Hefner by the rise of AIDS and the moral majority. Some have suggested that these factors combined to precipitate the collapse of Hef's chain of clubs and a drop in circulation of the magazine. They have also suggested that the resulting pressure triggered Hef's stroke in 1985.

In retrospect, Hefner wishes he hadn't remained silent while under attack by Bogdanovich. He might have been able to soften the blows delivered in the damning press stories the attack instigated. "The implication was that when Paul Snider killed

Dorothy he was doing what the typical reader of *Playboy* was doing when he looked at the magazine's pictures," says an incensed Hefner, who rips the Diet Pepsi label off his bottle while discussing this period. "Now that is an agenda which is just so sick. I remember listening to a radio interview with [feminist and Bogdanovich ally] Andrea Dworkin at the time in which she said that pornography kills. One listener called in and asked for an example, and Dworkin simply said 'Dorothy Stratten,' but she wouldn't elaborate." Hef concedes that he had never felt so wounded or dehumanized in his life. "People have called me a lot of things over the years, but never dishonest," he says. "Gee, even as a kid, they called me Honest Hugh." But things often work themselves out in strange ways. The new millennium brought Hef a rapprochement with Stratten's younger sister, who later married Bogdanovich. She is presently working part-time at the Playboy Mansion. As for Bogdanovich, the only time Hef sees him these days is on the tube; the director plays a shrink on the hit series *The Sopranos*. The irony of Bogdanovich's role has not escaped Hef.

The moral millionaire approves of the job Bill Clinton did as president, but not necessarily of his comportment in the Oral Office. "He just couldn't keep his pants on. The fact that it didn't hurt his approval rating, however, reflects changing social values." Then Hef muses, "I guess my only real problem with the president is that I wish he had better taste. You can get the boy into the White House, but you can't get the Arkansas out of the boy. What is unique about Clinton is not that he fucked around, but that he felt a lot of guilt related to it. He's still a good Baptist boy at heart — it's a very American conflict."

Whereas Clinton might be nursing a few regrets, Hef has none. Life, he says, "is a dangerous game. I've seen lots of tragedy. I've lost some very dear friends. I've made some business mistakes. Of course, you'd like to be able to change some things, but if you did, what else would change?" He is the first to admit that his magazine has taken a beating. In its heyday, in the seventies, *Playboy* sold seven million copies a month. Now it's down to three million. Hef attributes this decline to competition from T.V., video, and the Internet — some of which is generated by his own companies. And there's also a distribution problem. Convenience and drug stores throughout North America won't handle adult magazines anymore. "There has even been a controversy about taking an issue of *Cosmo* off the racks because they thought the cover was just too sexy," Hef giggles. "Yet, with all this, we continue to be the biggest-selling, most influential men's magazine in America. Yeah, we've dropped from first place to first place."

And women still line up to appear in *Playboy* pictorials. "You see that whenever we do the college issues and we get thousands of women who audition. And it's not like there's much money involved, either. It's become a source of celebrity. But part of the motivation is that the negative implications of nudity have disappeared in many quarters." Just ask Pamela Anderson and Jenny McCarthy, whose careers soared after they appeared in the buff in *Playboy*. Or ask Darva Conger, the not-so-shy *Who Wants to Marry a Multi-Millionaire* winner who bared all to extend her moment of notoriety. The mention of Conger's failed marriage to her *Who Wants to Marry a Multi-Millionaire* Mr. Wrong causes Hef to rethink his assertion that he's free of regrets. On second thought, he wouldn't take the marriage tumble again. "I'd still like to come back as me," he reflects, "but, truly, marriage does something to a relationship. It tends to make people take one another for granted. All I will say is that the major justification for marriage is children." His two sons, Marston and Cooper, live with their mom, Kimberly, in an estate adjoining the Playboy Mansion. "The interesting thing is that Kimberly and I are now closer than when we were married."

What would seem to be the pivotal moment in Hef's life occurred in the early fifties. He was toiling as a promotion copywriter at *Esquire* in Chicago for sixty dollars a week when the magazine moved its operations to New York. Hef's request for a five-dollar raise was rejected, so he decided to stay put and start his own magazine. And the rest is, as they say, history. This, however, wouldn't necessarily be Hef's pick as pivotal moment. That came much earlier. "When I was a small boy," he confides, "I had a blanket that had bunny rabbits on it. I called it my bunny blanket and I kept it on my bed. I had a mastoid operation when I was about six. When I was recovering, my parents bought me a dog. He slept in a box next to my bed. But the dog got sick, so I put my bunny blanket on him to keep him warm. The dog only lived a couple of weeks. When he died, they took my bunny blanket away and burned it." Hef is misty-eyed. "So I was determined back then to create a Bunny empire." Citizen Kane back off.

Empire building remains all the rage in Los Angeles. But no matter how shrewd an entrepreneur you are, finding a new niche in which to launch your undertaking can be exasperating. For most people, but not all. Out here in the Lotusland there lives an enterprising woman who has borrowed a leaf or two from Hef's survival book. She has learned that little beats an old-fashioned licking when it comes to accumulating an old-fashioned fortune — and keeping your mate's machine ticking.

I came too soon. Could I have committed any greater faux-pas when dealing with one of America's most renowned sex educators? Can you feel my shame? But Lou Paget, the Calgary-born sexpert who shot to prominence through her Frankly Speaking Sexuality Seminars, is remarkably understanding. After all, she has heard every imaginable excuse over the course of her fifteen years in the boudoir-satisfaction business. I try to explain to Paget that my hotel doorman told me it would take fifteen minutes by cab to reach her Beverly Hills abode. It took five. Never, ever, arrive early for a meeting of any kind with a lady, Paget gently chides. Though she dispenses advice about tenderness in the sack, the perky, redheaded Paget, with her authoritative (though awfully seductive) voice, evokes memories for me of the kindly school librarian who tried to keep me in line during my formative years.

And coming too soon is only the first gaffe I will commit on this day. I'll soon make the mistake of assuming that Lou is short for Louise, but I am quickly informed that the name is actually an abbreviation for Linda Lou, which is a handle that conjures up a dim bimbo cousin of Li'l Abner, which is precisely what I blurt out to Paget, because my self-edit button is obviously malfunctioning today.

Despite the fame and fortune she's derived from those seminars and from two hot-selling opuses, *How to Be a Great Lover* and *How to Give Her Absolute Pleasure*, Paget lives in a surprisingly compact apartment in one of the more modest sections of Beverly Hills. In fact, her place could belong to a librarian, what with all the family photos scattered about the living room and the cute fridge magnets that anchor reminders of upcoming rendezvous. My first inkling that Paget isn't the school-librarian type comes when I glimpse what's inside her dishwasher. No cups or plates in this load. Only latex phalluses. White, black, and mulatto, in a variety of sizes. Then, in a corner of her living room I spot a box of goodies that wouldn't likely belong to a librarian, either. These items make up Paget's line of products: the space-age vibrator, the Magic Ring, Jelly Thai Beads, and Love Gum — a full-potency gum for romantics with a dietary supplement and ginseng.

Oh, and did I neglect to mention that Paget has acquired additional fame by teaching Hollywood A-list actresses and the wives of Hollywood A-list studio execs — among scores of other grateful women who also wish to remain anonymous — the finer points of fellatio? A few times a week, Paget packs a briefcase with dildos and makes her way to the Beverly Hills Holiday Inn. Awaiting her are groups of ten to fifteen women, each of whom has happily shelled out $150 to be enlightened by Paget. Opening her briefcase, Paget invites her students to select their weapons. These they stick to plates, and the lesson begins.

Paget shows the women how to do the Penis Samba, which involves coordinating the hands with the mouth and which, if done well, will apparently make the male organ dance. The Ode to Bryan requires some deft hand-crossing; Basket Weaving is executed with cupped hands. And, of course, there's the Heartbeat of America, which can allegedly bring the dead back to life. What a sight to behold: all these studious women sucking and licking and laughing. School was never like this before. But it's not all blowjobs. Paget also demonstrates the Italian Method, whereby the woman puts a condom on her man's penis without using her hands. According to Paget, you don't have to be Houdini to roll a condom on with your mouth.

In her apartment, sitting on a love seat, Paget exudes the serenity of someone who knows that she has performed an extraordinary public service. Thousands of contented customers can't all be wrong. She has now widened her base of operations and conducts seminars throughout the United States and Canada. And in L.A. she has initiated a monthly seminar for men who are curious to see what Paget's female students have been clamoring about. According to the lore, Paget picked up pointers on fellatio from a gay male friend, who liked to use a latte spoon as a demonstration tool. That was back in the late eighties. Since then, Paget, forty-four, has compiled even more relevant info.

Paget's strength, apart from her dazzling instructional technique, is that she never blushes. Nor does she have any misgivings about what she does. "I wasn't raised Catholic or Jewish, so I know nothing from guilt," she says, flashing an enormous smile. "But I was raised by a mother who was raised by a real Victorian." Alas, incentive. Calgary wasn't big enough or progressive enough to satisfy her dreams, and the same could be said about her then-hubby. So she bailed out of the city and the marriage and headed for California — La-La Land, circa 1989. "California is user-friendly for people," she says. "And L.A. in particular allows people their idiosyncrasies. The city supports new thinking and encourages people to explore their sexuality and their lifestyles in general." In other words, Paget and L.A. were made for one another.

By the bye, Paget wants us to know that she never employs fruits or vegetables in her classrooms, despite what a few published reports have suggested. It's strictly latex. It's also strictly confidential. Paget won't divulge the identity of her students. She won't even put their real names in her computer. Not even her agent or her identical twin sister in Toronto, with whom she shares everything, has a clue who Paget's illustrious students are. Which probably explains why the redhead from Calgary is still in business. Many in her position would have sold their client lists to the highest bidder long ago — perhaps one of the supermarket tabs — but not Paget. She just sees herself as someone who disseminates info that everyone needs and should want.

Okay, so a technique called the Taffy Pull may be hard to swallow, but it does result in instant gratification. Guaranteed. "Students have said to me that their hands have been attached to their bodies their whole lives but that they were never aware what they could do with them prior to the seminars," Paget says. "Now that makes me feel really good." Yet Paget is the first to admit that she's had no formal sex training. She has never attempted to pass herself off as a therapist. "I just know that there's more out there than people are aware of."

Her catharsis came when she was leaving the driveway of the Calgary home she'd shared with her husband. "Something was missing in my life, and I couldn't put my finger on it." That something was a solid sexual relationship. "It had been at best ho-hum. But my thinking was: Why bother doing something unless you do it really well?" So, drawing on her University of Calgary degree in physical sciences with a major in biology, and indulging her "insatiable curiosity," Paget attempted to learn all she could about sex.

After scouring the porn videos and mags, she came to a conclusion. Much of the adult material available was geared exclusively to men. "They were only forgetting about fifty percent of the population, that's all. Then the books I read would tell me stuff that wasn't always practical. I wasn't getting the nuts and bolts. I wanted to know, where are people putting their fingers, toes, and tongues?" So Paget started asking her friends where they put their fingers, toes, and tongues, and they would invariably look at her like she'd been smoking (what they are fond of calling in Calgary) some of that "wacky tabacky." Eventually, though, they opened up; so did friends of friends, and many told Paget that men consistently missed the G-spot with their flickering tongues. "Tell them to suck on us the way we suck on them," several women advised Paget. But it wasn't a one-way street. Pag heard men complain of women licking up the wrong tree. "We're all born with the ability to vocalize, but it doesn't mean we can instantly speak English," she says. Paget's point is that everything requires learning and that open communication is paramount, particularly when it comes to the delicate arts of fellatio and cunnilingus.

Paget is still incredulous when she recounts the case of the middle-aged couple who came to her in search of a solution to the husband's impotence. The problem turned out to be that neither partner moved during sex. They waited and waited and waited for something to happen and, without fail, the man would falter. "They never knew what to do," Paget says with a sigh. "If no one tells you, how do you know? And if you're too shy to ask, how can anyone help?"

Obviously, many people have been left in the dark, or Paget wouldn't be doing the boffo business she does. "I just can't believe the number of guys I've encountered who think that all they have to do is ram it in hard and the woman is instantly satisfied. Yowsers, no!" She shakes her head. "I see my role now as being a 'consumer report' on sexuality. The stuff is out there, but it has never been put together cohesively. I have a different way of explaining a sensitive subject to people, and they are getting it."

Paget says that the number one rule for giving great head is actually to employ great hand technique. "The men who are best at oral sex use every part of their faces," she continues. "And did you know that a man requires a smooth lower lip if he is to give maximum pleasure while kissing or heading south of the border? Oh yes, the woman is like the most complicated fuse box in the house. If you put too much circuit in too quickly to an area before it's ready, you'll either blow the mental fuse or the physical fuse." She ain't just referring to fellatio.

Once we get onto the topic of dos and don'ts, Paget wants to emphasize that most women detest it when their nipples are pinched. "Guys get programmed by porn flicks, where they see women going crazy after getting their nipples pinched. But in the real world it doesn't work like that. Women have to be relaxed before. Then they might go for it later. For women, you see, so much of sex is so mental. You have to seduce their minds before you work on their bodies." Another no-no: inserting your tongue in a woman's ear. "If you really want to know, it makes us feel like our head is in the dishwasher," Paget exclaims. "Women prefer tenderness to the sides of their ears and necks. Men, on the other hand, like ear action. The male ear is a strong sex receptor."

Paget finds that she often, and unwittingly, assumes the role of sexual traffic cop during her seminars. Women participants will compare notes with other women and then seek Paget's definitive ruling. She does her best to keep her sessions from becoming male bash-a-thons. "I am so over male-bashing jokes," she says. "If you substituted women or Afro-Americans, they would be entirely inappropriate. The seminars are simply designed to expand the buffet." It's no accident, then, that many of Paget's analogies relate to eating. "Sometimes you want breakfast, sometimes hors d'oeuvres, or sometimes the whole meal deal. But sex, one way or another, is what keeps people connected."

Demand for Paget's seminars has never been greater, and she has been conducting them since 1996. What intrigues her, and others, is that this success has not been dependent upon advertising. Paget hasn't done any. Appropriately, it's all been word of mouth. Speaking of word of mouth, Paget denies reports that she practices what she preaches too frequently. "If I did a quarter of what people said I did, I'd have no time to do anything else. People can say I'm sleazy if they want, but like I told my father, the books and seminars are not based on me, but rather based on what I've learned."

Paget does admit that, when their schedules permit, she's been seeing an unnamed talk-show host who's based back East. Inquiring minds want to know: Is this man content? Paget slaps me on the knee and giggles, "Oh, you're such a guy. I'm sure people are thinking that when I'm in a relationship I have got this 'Hey baby, I'm amazing!' attitude. Well, that's not me." Still, Paget does concede that she and her gentleman suitor share a "strong connection." "Great," sez I, "but tell me, please, Ms. Paget, that the guy is not Jerry Springer." She assures me he isn't.

Keeping herself up-to-date on health issues relating to sex is a priority for Paget. "Sex must be fun, but it must be, above all, safe. I'm smart enough to know what I don't know, so I ask medical experts and they tell me we could be on the brink of a major global health crisis if we don't watch ourselves."

Curiously, Paget has never encountered hostility from feminists. "I think of myself as a feminist. But, no, I've never had any feminist attack me. If they did, I would challenge them. After all, what I teach gives women the most natural access to the most powerful part of themselves — their sexuality." Perhaps it's a testament to changing attitudes, but a decade or so back Paget would have faced plenty of resistance when trying to get her seminars off the ground. "Times have grown up. Time has taken a dose of reality," she says. "We can no longer ignore sexual culture and we can't ignore relationships culture, especially at a time when humans are maturing faster than ever and there is more information than ever out there."

Gazing into her crystal ball, Paget sees sex of the future as being more of a celebration than it has been to date. People will be more tolerant than ever. "There is nothing that will validate someone's sexuality more than being accepted as they are and not being judged, whether that person prefers straight missionary sex, cybersex, being a swinger, or wanting to be a virgin until they are married. At least I've helped make people aware that there are different ways to talk about sex and do it." This is all a far cry from the old days, when sex was either not discussed in public or dealt with through humor. Paget notes that "the Eskimos have a gazillion words for snow. One day, maybe we'll have a gazillion words for sex."

The pit bull of comedy already has a gazillion words for sex. He also has a Jack Russell terrier and a wife and a twelve-year-old daughter on whom he dotes. He lives in a quaint bungalow on Sunnyside Avenue in the quaint oceanfront community of Marina Del Rey. He buys his audio, video, and computer equipment at a store called The Good Guys in his suburban 'hood. At the moment, however, Bobby Slayton has little time to chat. He's planning a Mother's Day picnic at the beach with his minibrood. Catering arranged, there's pressing business to deal with. He has an auction to attend. On his computer. Slayton bids for tchotchkes on E-Bay. He loves to collect stuff. He has an autographed baseball from the 1960 New York Yankees, bearing the signatures of Mickey Mantle, Roger Maris, and Yogi Berra, no less. He also has a battalion of vintage pinball machines.

I'm confused. Actually, I'm concerned. Has the nastiest man in comedy gone mellow? Slayton attempts to reassure me. He proudly points to the replicas of the *Creatures from the Black Lagoon* that are festooned around his office. He shows off an ashtray from the Bates Motel (you know, *Psycho*). A really creepy skeleton-clown drawing created by serial murderer John Wayne Gacy. A replica of John Dillinger's death mask. An Andy Warhol litho of an electric chair. An autographed photo of Boris Karloff. A family photo, of sorts, featuring himself and daughter Natasha cavorting with *Nightmare on Elm Street*'s Freddy Kreuger. And, a really scary artifact: a ten thousand dollar cash-advance agreement, dated 1950, that's made out to, and signed by, Dean Martin and Jerry Lewis. "Still think I've softened and turned normal?" Slayton screams. "No insult intended, but guess not," I reply. "Sorry to have ever doubted you."

Slayton and I hop into the family sedan and tool down the beach road to Hermosa. Slayton is headlining tonight at the Comedy and Magic Club, where Jay Leno does a regular Sunday evening gig to try out his *Tonight Show* spiel on regulars who just can't get enough of the man during the week. But Jay Leno can't boast that the club posts warnings to prospective clients about the nature of his act. Bobby Slayton can. This, I've never seen before. Yellow flyers are plastered all over the club's entrance: "Warning! The Headlining Performer this evening, Bobby Slayton, may be found offensive, antagonistic, controversial, crude, graphic, vulgar, and politically incorrect to many! If you are faint at heart, you may want to reconsider!"

Talk about a brilliant marketing strategy. The joint is packed. The pit bull is sporting an ear-to-ear grin. And why not? Strangely enough, he, too, is considered to be at the vanguard of the ever-mutating sexual revolution, and Slayton is quick to point out that there are few more revolting — or funny — than him. But before he can shock the troops, opening attraction and fellow lewd boy Nick Griffith takes the stage and loosens up the audience. "Just read in some scientific journal that Prozac inhibits ejaculation. That'll cheer you up," Griffith ruminates. "Of course, if you can't ejaculate, all your other problems do pale by comparison." Griffith also has a word of warning for all the ladies in the house, and despite the fact that this is a night of nasty comedy, the women outnumber the men. There is, as is fast becoming evident, a new phenomenon sweeping the land. The thrust of sexual politics is changing. "If your boyfriend doesn't think your breasts are big enough . . . change boyfriends. Don't get your breasts enlarged . . . get a midget. He'll think your breasts are big enough." Then Griffith makes an unusual analogy: "A bisexual girlfriend . . . that's the Swiss Army knife of women."

Now it's Slayton's turn. He flies onto the stage. The subject is premature ejaculation. His wife, he insists, has told him that he should see a specialist about this condition. Slayton is undaunted. "Why?" he bellows. "It's your problem!" Slayton has a confession to make. "Valentine's Day. Mother's Day. Where's my day? I want Blowjob Day. But, no, all I've got is Palm Sunday. Palm Monday. Palm Tuesday . . ." Appearances on the homefront notwithstanding, Slayton has a low threshold for romance. *Titanic* made him puke, but *The Hand That Rocks the Cradle* — now that was a flick. "Babysitter comes over and tries to kill the wife and fuck the husband. Can't find help like that anymore." At the conclusion of his set, Slayton spots a family in the crowd. "Sir, your kids learned a lot this evening. That you can get up on stage and say 'Fuck' and not go to college and still make a great living."

The crowd eats it all up. Among the applauding spectators is one Melissa Monet. Her name doesn't ring a bell? Well, you may remember her from such cinematic adventures as *Bad Girls 3* or *Strap On Sally 5*. Monet was a major blue movie star until she moved behind the camera and started directing. She also did the doc *Porn: It's a Living*. Monet liked calling the shots so much that now she's directing flicks that feature fully clothed humans. But Monet has no regrets about her stint in porno. Far from it.

Over brunch the next day at a homey Venice Beach café, the brash, petite brunette with the alluring eyes takes a swipe at those who get all sanctimonious about the adult-film industry. "There are as many fucked-up people at IBM as there are in porn — maybe more." Monet doesn't hold back. A transplanted New Yorker, she's as tough as nails. Her father is Italian Catholic and her mother is German Jewish. Orthodox Jewish, in fact. "Sure, there are some pathetic people in porno. But there's a real dichotomy. The world doesn't want to know that the majority of the people in porn aren't sick, fucked up, and twisted. I will always remember the great times. I look at other people sitting around in their do-nothing, go-nowhere jobs, and I couldn't be more thrilled that I took the path I did."

Working on a stack of peanut butter pancakes, Monet declares that times have changed in the porn world. The *Boogie Nights* days of the late seventies and early eighties have given way to an era of relative moderation and reflection. She has encountered people from all walks of life, she claims, and finds that the porn scene has a high concentration of informed and interesting members. She is referring to the likes of actor/director John Leslie and AVN publisher Paul Fishbein, but she holds a special place in an unspecified body part for *Screw*'s Al Goldstein. Porn Renaissance man and activist Bill Margold doesn't fare so well in Monet's estimation. "He talks the good talk, but doesn't always walk the good walk."

As a child, Monet dreamed of becoming a ballerina or a marine biologist. Her hero was — and still is — underwater explorer Jacques Cousteau. She played classical trumpet in high school. She attended a yeshiva. She had a bat mitzvah. She never caught the acting bug — "I had the greed bug"; this led her to work as an accountant after finishing high school, but she rapidly became bored with the straight life. At nineteen, she made a unique career move. She took a job as a sex surrogate, entering the convergence of the psychology and prostitution domains. The work was lucrative, and Monet felt that she was performing a humanitarian service. "I was teaching people how to fix their sexual problems and I was having lots of sex as a means of teaching. I studied Masters and Johnson as well as *The Hite Report*. It was legit, to a certain extent. We helped clients. But we bilked them, too. Then again, people were happy to pay anything for help. Those were the days when there were no quick fixes. There was no Viagra then."

The on-the-job sex was almost never satisfying for Monet, but the goal was to assist others. "Fortunately, I was always into sex. When I was five, I became aware of sex. I didn't know what I was doing, but I had lots of fun exploring. I had to keep my interest in sex hidden, though. My parents were the Cleavers, highly educated professionals with very high moral standards. It wasn't until I was thirty that they actually found out what I had been up to all those years. But what could they do then?" Monet has her own set of moral standards. She has zero tolerance for child pornography. She feels that those who exploit children should suffer the severest penalties. "A lot of the people in the business have children and are more strict and protective towards them than regular types. They're very careful about what their kids can watch on T.V. It's almost like a double standard."

Monet didn't last long as a sex surrogate. She soon switched to the highly rewarding field of escort servicing. Only one problem: "I wasn't getting a lot of calls, because for the only period in my life I was fat." She ended up working the phones for the escort service, and by doing so she found her niche. She learned the ropes and started running the service herself. She was making more money than she had ever dreamed possible, and she was all of twenty one at the time. But the hours were long, and the strain took its toll; Monet came down with pneumonia. So, back to the straight world she went to toil nine-to-five as a bookkeeper. "As soon as I got there I remembered why I had given up this world in the first place. Sometimes you need a catalyst to remind yourself of what kind of life you want to lead. And there was no way I was going to spend my life rotting in some desk job." There would be no more turning back. Monet resumed answering the escort agency's phones. One day, an "interesting" call came in, and since no escort was available, Monet took the job herself. "I was thin again, and made a shitload of money on that job. It wasn't hard work. I could handle the customers. My time as a sex surrogate gave me a great education on dealing with people and I was up to speed on safe sex."

Eventually, Monet was enticed into working at a high-end brothel by one of Manhattan's most renowned madames. There, she learned all about fashion and food. She learned how to talk to corporate players and dress for any occasion. Polished, and open to almost anything, Monet was in demand. Then she got an offer she couldn't refuse. A client offered to pay her fifty thousand dollars for three hours of work, which didn't entail sleeping with him. "He just wanted to watch another girl spank me. It was an odd situation. I had never even been spanked as a child. So I wasn't prepared. And let me tell you that after five hundred spanks, I was plenty sore. But it just goes to show what sort of proclivities some people have. This was a wealthy businessman whose photo was forever in the *Wall Street Journal*, and this is what excited him more than anything in the world. All I kept saying to myself as the other girl was slapping me was 'k-ching, k-ching, k-ching.'"

Monet stops reminiscing for a moment when she sees a friend passing by, pushing her newborn baby in a stroller. The friend stops, and Monet prattles babytalk and plays with the infant. She adores children and dogs. "Just because I was a dominatrix doesn't mean I'm not sensitive," she cracks. When the baby and her mother head off to the beach, Monet tucks back into her pancakes and her memories. After observing her madame on the job, Monet decided that she wanted to be her own boss. She bought a book of numbers from another madame, and, at age twenty-five, she found herself running a brothel that rivaled Manhattan's finest. She was being compared to the Mayflower Madame, Sydney Biddle Barrows. She was living in a luxurious carriage house. She was being wined and dined by corporate and showbiz players. And she was stockpiling enough cash to retire to Hawaii. Which is precisely what she did. She cashed in her chips and became a surfer. She got a tan. She ate well. She eschewed alcohol, tobacco, and drugs. "I became a professional designated driver," she quips. In about a year, Monet had blown her savings. "Actually, it was the guy whom I was supporting who blew my fortune for me." Love is strange.

Despite it all, however, Monet is an incurable romantic. She never engages in one night stands. Her relationships are long-term, intense, and often turbulent. "I get too mushy and, consequently, I get into problems. And this is as a result of dating regular guys. The biggest mistake I ever made in my life was dating a customer. I did that only once and it was disastrous."

Monet still had "mushy" feelings for the beau who'd cleaned out her bank account. When he decided that they should relocate to California, where he would make his fortune in the porno biz, she agreed. "Sadly, he was lacking the necessary equipment for the job," Monet recalls. "I didn't have the heart to tell him. But all the porn casting agents laughed when he displayed his wares. He didn't get it. And here I am sitting in the offices, holding his hand, and the agents are asking me if I want in. And I'm thinking, 'This is the only thing in the sex business I haven't done, so why not?'"

For a brief spell, Monet had bought into the bungalow-and-white-picket-fence dream, but after this experience she realized that such scenarios weren't for her. Saying goodbye to her deficient beau, she said hello to a brand-new life — as porno queen Melissa Monet. Although close to thirty when she entered the biz, Monet made more than one hundred movies and was nominated for several porno Oscars in less than three years. "It was a terrific ride at first, and like anything else, it tapered off when I was no longer the new girl. But it only hit home after I was doing a scene with a woman and I realized that I had shorts older than she was."

Monet is proud of her scruples. "I never did anal or gang-bangs. It was always one-on-one. But ultimately sex was a means to an end. I was a performer. Of course, women are mostly great actresses. That's because few enjoy sex." Because Monet could ride a motorcycle as well as perform on her back, side, and tummy, she got a bonus and did *Strap-On Sally 5* and 6. She worked with Ron Jeremy and Mr. Marcus, Amanda Adams and Careena Collins. "I've only met two or three people in the business I could choke. Guys who couldn't get laid in a whorehouse with a fistful of thousands. Misogynist bigots and freaks who should rot in hell. Plus, they were racists and anti-Semites." But tell us how you really feel, Melissa. "These types," explains

Monet, "made me realize that I had to get onto the other side of the camera." Her first foray into directing was for an adult CD-Rom. "I watched all of three movies and figured I could direct. I fucked up, but it came out okay. Then I watched other directors. And I asked a lot of questions. And I learned, because I am a sponge and I'm smart." She would go on to direct, produce, and write close to fifty films for the Spice Channel. She would also direct a few erotica features for mainstream pay T.V. One day during this period, while she was walking her dog on the beach, she met another dog owner and they started discussing life. When Monet confessed that she had been a porno star, "The woman was shocked. She asked what a nice girl like me was doing in a business like that. Then she ran away. I yelled that I wasn't raping, pillaging, or killing. She wouldn't listen. I was upset." Inspired by this incident, Monet embarked upon a new project — the documentary film *Porn: It's a Living*. She wanted to convey to others what the business and the people who inhabit it are really like.

These days, she's directing a series of straight comedies and producing a straight feature, in which Ron Jeremy has been cast, for once, in a small part. Plus, she writes health and fitness columns under a pseudonym for various health magazines. "Whatever floats your boat, I say. Everybody in the porno business has dreams of crossing over into so-called legit movies. It's boredom. But it's also the fact that if you put on five pounds, you're being offered gang-bangs for two hundred dollars. It's like anything. You have to keep your wits about you. It's not easy. You have to persevere. That's why I'm so proud of myself."

These days, also, Monet yearns for a stable romance. "I want someone who will really understand me. But then I'm thinking that the kind of guy who will really understand me is some twisted fuck, and I don't want him sharing my bed. It's a bit of a dilemma." That it is. In the meantime, Monet's closest companion remains her dog — a pit bull. That's right, Mr. Nasty, Bobby Slayton, has a Jack Russell; and Melissa Monet, porno tenderheart, has a pit bull. Hmm. Monet, however, sees no irony in this. She insists that not only are the ladies of porn tougher than the guys, but they are also poised to take over the business of sex. Furthermore, she says, the ladies of New York City, her hometown, are the toughest of them all. "Check it out," Monet dares me.

Chapter 3

BITE ME!
THE BIG
APPLE

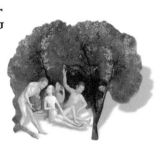

"You are really some kind of stupid moron," the scowling bartender tells the gentleman perched on the stool. "Don't *ever* place a paper napkin next to a candle! You could burn the whole place down, asssssshole!" Yet the chastened patron seems relieved. "He got off easy," explains Christine O'Day, manager of the establishment. "Yeah, he got verbally abused but good — plus, he didn't have to pay for it."

Wow, does it get any better than this? Evidently not, for the well-heeled clients of La Nouvelle Justine. Located on Second Street in New York's funky East Village, this place bills itself as the original S&M café. Since 1996, people have flocked here to order a rum punch — which is often just that. Apart from the haute-cuisine nibbles and an array of exotic cocktails, they come — literally and figuratively — for an old-fashioned spanking or some doggy-like obedience training or merely a little public humiliation, like the tongue lashing the gent at the bar received. Unlike this fella, though, most have to pony up at least twenty dollars for the privilege of being abused by one of the staff's shapely, though surly, dominatrixes.

It's a week night at La Nouvelle Justine. O'Day doubts that it will fill up this evening. The place relies heavily on the young yuppie trade. "As much as they would like it and deserve it, they don't generally have the time to get spanked during the week," O'Day says with a shrug. Fortunately, the café is able to subsist on bachelor and bachelorette parties during the week. Last night, the members of a young women's softball team were given the kind of thrashing they never get on the field, and they paid dearly for the privilege. Drinks and food set them back a whack of cash. So did the floggings. Then they stocked up on the souvenir spiked dogcollars and dildos from the display shelf at the end of the bar.

Still, O'Day has certain doubts about her clientele. "They are more voyeurs and poseurs than real fetishists," she says. "If they're not really juiced, they don't quite grasp the concept that they must pay to be spanked or humiliated by one of our dominatrixes. Duh!" As she speaks, in walks this evening's party of unsuspecting bachelorettes, a group of twenty-four women from the high-stress field of high-tech recruiting. Each one is an attractive twentysomething who earns a six-figure salary. Adventurous though these women may be, they've never set foot in an S&M café before, but they're open to new challenges and they do love to drink. Says one group member, Andrea, "I'm not knowingly into abusing or being abused, but that could quickly change." Adds her buddy Liz: "If it works out some of the aggression I must deal with during the day, it could be a blast."

The ladies concur that times have changed in the corporate world. In days gone by, it would have been the boys letting off steam in an afterhours strip club while the girls (and they want to impress upon me that there weren't many of their kind in upper-level positions in the old days) snuggled up to a good book. "Not that there's anything wrong with reading," says Andrea. "But we need to unwind, too, and get wild. So we go to an S&M café to bond with the girls." And what better place to bond than a fashionable, dungeon-like environment where bondage is on the menu. Andrea concludes that it's not much of a stretch for them to venture from their workplace to the world of La Nouvelle Justine: "We're brokers. What does that mean? We buy and sell people." Gazing at the overhead T.V. screen, the girls take in some black-and-white fifties nudie flicks that feature submissive ladies in revealing lingerie. Finally they notice the spanking cage with the whipping post, to which handcuffed clients are chained.

Forever the pessimist, manager O'Day still doesn't have high hopes for this lot. A former dominatrix whose arms are covered with macabre tattoos, O'Day, attired in regulation rubber, will, in a pinch, fill in with some inspired flogging. "The problem is that most of these types only volunteer to get whipped when they're drunk, so we have to wait. They're so paranoid, too. Then some actually think we'll pay them to dominate us. Really! How do they think we survive? That makes me so mad that I want to whip them even harder." She rolls her eyes in disgust. "What planet do some of these people come from, anyway?" But the customers of La Nouvelle Justine do learn quickly that they are rarely right — and they learn to like that. O'Day estimates that one in two comes back for more abuse. "It's a good thing," she remarks. "Every restaurant needs regulars in order to survive."

While the high-tech recruiting girls have their dinner, I sit at the bar. The bartender, still scowling, casts me a dismissive glance and barks, "Who the hell are you?" "That's more like it," I answer. I don't want to feel left out of the abuse. This bartender, whose name is Mistress Otter, just sneers. She is perfect for the part. Her garish eye makeup could qualify her for the role of Morticia Addams. Then again, Morticia would never sport a skin-tight vinyl swimsuit like Mistress Otter's. And it's probably just a coincidence that there's a primer on the Heimlich maneuver posted behind the bar. "Mistress Otter, you wouldn't choke a customer, would you?" Mistress Otter does what Mistress Otter does best. She sneers.

Meanwhile, O'Day is stocking the bar with lace-up boots,

each containing a champagne bottle. "I guess you could say we're a novelty restaurant," she says. Mistress Otter mutters something incomprehensible. It's worth noting that La Nouvelle Justine is owned by the same gent who runs Lucky Cheng's, an adjoining café that specializes in transvestite karaoke — clearly a novelty, as well.

The recruiters are ignoring the no smoking sign posted behind them. I point this out to Mistress Otter. She, of course, sneers. "Ah, civil disobedience," I say. "That's a good thing, right?" Mistress Otter — well, she's not amused by anything I say, so I busy myself studying my surroundings. The decor, apart from the whipping cage, is comprised of posters of babes in bondage. Strewn along the bar are specialty mags, like the latest issue of Mistress Otter's fave, *Bizarre Rubber*. I'm soon bored with leafing through *Bizarre Rubber*, so I take a chance. I ask Mistress Otter if I might peruse a menu, for I'm a little hungry. She looks ready to shove one of those leather-booty champagne bottles into one of my orifices, but she resists and thrusts a menu in my direction instead. As I expected, the menu reflects the theme of the establishment: Calamari au Marquis de Sade, Salade de Punishments, Mistress Canard, Guillotine Crevettes. Mistress Otter indicates that if I had any taste, and she's pretty darned certain that I don't, I would order the Mistress Canard — no relation to Mistress Otter I am informed in no uncertain terms. "It's a duck dish, you assssshole!" she spits at me. "I know," I tell her. "Well, there's a surprise," she shoots back. "All the same, I don't like your attitude." Mistress Otter could get Mike Tyson eating out of her hand, or a reasonable facsimile.

The bachelorette recruiters are getting antsy. They are also getting pissed. They demand more drinks from Mistress Otter, who doesn't take kindly to receiving orders from corporate gals. She spills a couple of drinks. She is mighty steamed. I refrain from initiating more idle conversation and thus avoid a swat to the lower extremities. Manager O'Day is starting to take exception to the loudness of the conversation emanating from the girls' table. She is nursing a hangover. "I'm going to have to go over there and slap them down, if they don't behave," she says. Which, ironically, is her job.

Mistress Otter takes time to create her specialty cocktail: a strawberry daiquiri served in a dog bowl. This seems to please her. But not for long. The hen party is starting to sing along, loudly and badly out of key, to "I Love Rock & Roll." Mistress Otter is prepared to pummel them for free; such is the extent of her displeasure. "If you don't stop singing, I'm gonna kick your asses," she screams, making it clear that she's not in the service business for the tips. "You all sing like shit!" O'Day also frowns as she surveys the scene. "These are the same people who normally give me dirty looks on the street. The beauty of it all, though, is that here I get to slap them around and get paid for it." She smiles. "And, let's face it. I couldn't work anywhere else but here. With my kind of attitude, I'd be fired in a minute." But, when it comes right down to it, O'Day and Mistress Otter are cynical for all the right reasons. It's their job. All this nastiness? It's no different than when a bunch of caffeinated football players get psyched up for a big game in the locker room.

"Everyday People" is now blasting through the speakers. Irony continues to abound. I point this out to Mistress Otter . . . Good grief! I've left my menu close enough to a candle that it starts to turn brown. Mistress Otter is beside herself. Before she can go ballistic, I attempt to apologize. To no avail. "You are so unbelievably stupid!" she hollers. "You could have burned the whole place down." "Thank you," I respond. "And is there a charge for the verbal abuse?" Mistress Otter is not sure whether she should answer or simply scratch my eyes out. Fortunately, she gets distracted by Mistress Debora, the resident dominatrix, who comes sauntering in wearing a smart leather bra-and-pants outfit and clutching a cat-o-nine-tails. Mistress Otter and Mistress Debora exchange pleasantries, of a sort. Mistress Debora then turns her attention to the singing recruiter girls, who are getting more plastered by the minute. "How are you all? No, what are you all?" The girls pay little heed to Mistress

Debora. This isn't a prudent course of action, because it makes Mistress Debora angry. She cracks her whip. "Shut the fuck up! Okay!" Now that she has their undivided attention, she tells them she's here to hurt them — for remuneration, to boot.

One of the girls leaves the table and approaches Mistress Debora by the bar. "Hold your horses," snaps Mistress Debora. "I'll talk to you when I'm good and ready." "But Mistress Debora," says the young recruiter, "one of the girls at the table has just gotten engaged and I think she deserves a really good spanking. What do you think?" Mistress Debora fires back, "Sit down until I'm ready. I hope to beat all your asses, after I numb them with drink."

As the girl retreats, Mistress Debora has a confession to make: "I can be such a bitch at times." Really? "Yes, but I can also be nice when the mood strikes." Mistress Debora allows that her line of work can be gratifying. "But it's a tough way to make a living. If I didn't have a couple of regular slaves come in for spankings, I'd be on welfare." Mistress Debora has another confession to make. She would like to have her own animal reserve, and she would spare the rod with the beasts that lived on it. "People can fuck off, but animals I love," she declares. She states that on a bad night in the whipping cage she'll make about sixty dollars. "On a good night, I'll make enough to pay the rent and buy beautiful fresh flowers the next day." For no apparent reason, Mistress Debora tells me that she's like a fine Italian wine — "getting better with age."

Even Mistresses Debora and Otter seem taken aback at what's happening over at the girls' table. Some of the more blitzed members of the group are undressing; they're displaying previously concealed tattoos to one another. "Amazing what a few drinks will do," Mistress Otter stammers with apparent disgust.

Let the games begin. Mistress Debora approaches the table like a stealthy tiger stalking her prey. The girls are not paying attention. Mistress Debora cracks her whip. Still they pay no attention. Mistress Debora makes a sudden grab for the boobs of a girl called Alexis. Mistress Debora now has their attention. Alexis makes a surprise admission: "If I had to choose between domination and submission, I'd choose to dominate. I feel like spankin' someone tonight." Alas, so does Mistress Debora. She settles instead for the perky Jewel, who has been busy showing off her tattoos. Mistress Debora cuffs Jewel to the cage and then blindfolds her. Jewel doesn't resist a bit. Alexis remarks that Jewel is "one of the most productive people in our company." Well, tonight her reward is getting her buttocks flogged. And she's enjoying it. Her coworkers, whooping it up at the table, are also enjoying it. Now Jewel is getting her derriere paddled and fondled by Mistress Debora, loving every minute of it. "Bet you won't like it if I make you lick my boots," Mistress Debora says to her. Well, Mistress Debora, for once, is dead wrong. Jewel licks her boots with relish.

Unshackled, her blindfold removed, Jewel makes her way to the bar for a drink. "That was just awesome," she says, her face flushed with excitement. "After a rough day at the office, there is no better feeling than getting spanked." So, Mistress Otter, did Jewel really enjoy herself?" I dare to ask. "Look at how red her face got. Did she enjoy it? Are you an idiot? She came. Duh!"

Next into the handcuffs is Kathy. Her crime: she just got engaged. While taking in the spectacle, Alexis observes that not so long ago few women would have volunteered to endure such abuse. "Times change," she says. "We're no longer afraid to explore different aspects of life. Believe it or not, getting whipped can be liberating." But hold that thought. All this talk and booze and abusive behavior is making Alexis crave a little action of her own. She asks Steve, the leather-garbed and otherwise genial waiter/busboy, if he'll submit to a flogging, for cash. He obliges, and Alexis flogs his fanny real good. "This is more fun than bowling night," Liz yelps. "And what a great way to get rid of all your frustrations." With genuine concern, Mistress Debora yells, "Hey, don't hit his balls! That could really hurt."

After she releases poor Steve from the whipping post, a

euphoric Alexis settles in at the bar. "It was such a release of tension," she enthuses. "I just can't explain how gratifying it all was. But it wasn't sexual. It was about power. The boys in the office can boast all they like, but they would be way too intimidated to submit to anything like this. They have images to protect, and they're not nearly as wild as they think they are." Mistress Otter commands Jewel to drink a Satanic Yoohoo cocktail from a doggy bowl. Jewel makes a mess. Mistress Otter orders her to clean it up. Jewel does what she is told. Alexis hands Steve a twenty-dollar bill and thanks him. "My pleasure, ma'am," he replies with appropriate subservience.

The girls are giggling and excited and really drunk now. No matter, Alexis says. "Most of the girls will never come back. I will, and I'm guessing Jewel will, but that's it." Jewel concurs: "Women are taking over. We're running businesses and calling the shots. And we just want to let loose." Jewel also confides, "I had been whipped before, but in the privacy of my friend's home. This was more of a thrill to get whipped in public." The one reservation Jewel has is that she feels Mistress Otter was a tad too frosty. To which the newly arrived Hedda Lettuce, the transvestite with the pencil-thin mustache, responds: "Honey, you want smiles? Go to McDonald's. But they're not going to whup your ass and they won't serve you drinks." Not yet, anyway. And McDonald's will never get a starring role in an S&M classic like *Tops and Bottoms* the way La Nouvelle Justine has. Mistresses Debora and Otter have commanded me to watch that flick all the way through — or else.

Voyeurs beware: *Tops and Bottoms*, shot on location around the Big Apple as well as other S&M capitals, offers little in the way of titillation. This documentary plunges viewers into the dungeon of sadomasochism, but its angle is far more academic than erotic. Indeed, *Tops and Bottoms*, while affording viewers a sometimes painful glimpse of S&M practices, sets out to prove the thesis that humankind's penchant for pain and submission stems from our hierarchal societal structures and our obsession with power. This sort of thinking doesn't strike a nerve in Mistresses Debora or Otter — nor in me, for that matter.

The documentary's director, Christine Richey, a native of Kingston, Ontario, and a self-described Canadian army brat, leaves many viewers cold with her simplistic, psychology / political science 101 theories regarding the assembly line and the notion that productivity is directly linked to the proliferation of dungeons and dominatrixes. However, when she gets off her podium and gives that capitalism-equals-bullwhips poppycock a rest, Richey, maker of the award-winning *In the Gutter and Other Good Places*, does deliver some fascinating insights into the history of S&M. She opens a window on people and places that few of us have ever encountered. She also manages to infiltrate a relationship between a sadist and masochist, providing us with the real skinny on the occasionally depraved human condition.

According to no less an authority than the Marquis de Sade, there is only one hierarchy in the world: tops and bottoms. Those who like to administer pain and / or sexual pleasure are the tops. Those who like to receive are the bottoms. Simple as that. With their wealth of experience backing them up, Mistresses Debora and Otter buy this thesis. De Sade was clearly a top; Leopold von Sacher-Masoch, however, was a bottom. A second-rate novelist, Masoch was not content with being humiliated by bad reviews. He also had an obsession with being pummeled senseless, preferably by his wife. He ended his days in an insane asylum. In 1886, Dr. Richard von Krafft-Ebing was able to blend the wisdom of de Sade and Masoch to identify a phenomenon he tagged "sadomasochism" — "a disturbance in the evolution of the psychosexual processes sprouting from the soil of psychical degeneration." Whatever gets you through the night.

It might not have had an official name, but S&M was with us long before de Sade, Masoch, and Krafft-Ebing hit the scene. In her film, Richey transports us back to the Middle Ages, when self-flagellation was all the rage and, apparently, served as an antidote to the Black Death and other such plagues. Then, Richey carries us forward to the repressive Victorian era, when protective parents would outfit their offspring with penis cages in order to ward off unwanted nocturnal emissions. According to Richey, the resultant angst may explain the fact that even de Sade's excesses paled by comparison to the floggings administered in the British public-school system. From here we goose-step into Nazi Germany, where we touch base with the ultimate psychotic sadist, Adolf Hitler. Unfortunately, Richey loses us when she leaps from Nazi Germany to the American corporate boardroom to New York's chic S&M restos, clubs, and dungeons — among them La Nouvelle Justine. The links are tenuous and our credulity is strained.

Richey then proceeds to jar us with a peek at the marriage of Robert and Mary Dange of Toronto. He is a former theater director. She has her PhD in cell biology and once conducted research at Toronto's Sick Children's Hospital. Both gave up their careers to work on their relationship and produce the S&M mag *Boudoir Noir*. Robert is a master. Mary is a slave. His pleasure is her pain, which, in turn, brings her pleasure. You get the picture. When we first encounter them, Robert and Mary have just signed a contract with an unsettled twenty-three-year-old university student called Mercedes. She has agreed to be Robert's slave, and he has agreed to punish her relentlessly. Things don't work out — Mercedes finds that she just can't get her jollies being whipped and tortured by Robert. She wants out. Robert feels betrayed. Some viewers may feel the urge to take a shower at this point. Some may also have arrived at the conclusion that the end of civilization is upon us.

So, I've watched *Tops and Bottoms* as I was commanded to do, but Mistresses Debora and Otter think I need further enlightenment. They order me to meet with one of Manhattan's (and, as such, the world's) most renowned whip ladies. Her name is Eva. Sweet, biblical, but watch your backside all the same, I'm cautioned.

Only the tongue is tied this morning. For most people, it would be far too early to chat about whips and chains and paddles and dungeons, but Eva Norvind, one of the galaxy's foremost authorities on fantasies featuring the aforementioned, is ready to ruminate on her favorite subject at any time. Not that anyone sipping coffee in this uptown hotel restaurant would ever guess that Norvind was once the Big Apple's dominatrix de choix. She isn't sporting spike heels or a slinky leather outfit. Clad in conservative gray slacks and matching top, Norvind looks almost matronly. These days, she's a psychosexual counselor, and the only thing she's flogging this morning is her life story, a documentary film titled *Didn't Do It for Love*.

Norvind has led a life, as they say. Born fifty-four years ago in Norway to a Russian prince and a Finnish sculptress, she danced in Europe and then made Westerns in Mexico. She obviously learned a thing or two about handling a lasso while engaged in the latter; that skill was put to good use in New York City, where she slipped with ease into the role of dominatrix. Although Norvind, who has a master's degree in human sexuality, says that she's since retired her whip, this instrument does come into play in the intriguing therapy operation she runs out of a posh Manhattan apartment. One room is for no-nonsense consultation; one is for computer studies; another is for crossdressers; and down the hall is a state-of-the-art dungeon, staffed with twenty-four dominatrixes, most of whom are women.

Dungeon clients pay from $250 (for an intern) to $500 an hour to be dominated and to explore their darker sides. At those prices, it's not surprising that most of Norvind's customers are from the city's upper crust: CEOs, judges, investment bankers, movie stars (none of whom she will name, of course). "Men in power need to surrender to bring balance to their lives," she explains.

Everything is above board in her dungeon, Norvind insists — which means that there is no sexual contact between staff members and the customers. For this reason, Norvind is permitted by New York state law to operate. "Our role is to help people who have sexual compulsions, fantasies that harm their lives and become financial burdens," she says matter-of-factly. "Then we try to help them find healthy outlets. I can relate. I'm a compulsive overeater." It all sounds so clinical that you might forget for a moment that Norvind makes a portion of her living from a medieval torture chamber where judges are led around on leashes and then spanked when they forget to heel. Bad judge.

But Norvind bristles — and feels like choking someone — when she hears about how the forces of justice fail to recognize the distinction between a dominatrix and a prostitute. One such case involved suburban-Toronto dominatrix Terri Jean Bradford, who was convicted and fined three thousand dollars for running a common bawdy house. Bradford argued that she'd done nothing felonious — unless using a flyswatter on an annoying law student who buzzed around her pad is a criminal act — and she vowed to continue cracking the whip. "All we're doing is helping submissive men with self-esteem problems," Norvind maintains. "It's about healing."

Norvind feels that most folks are conflicted because they're bombarded with sexual images, yet they are ruled by puritanical forces — a philosophy that curiously echoes Hugh Hefner's. "What is often lost is many sex offenders are that way because they can't enact their fantasies." She also suggests that legislators consider all the costs involved before trying to shackle another dominatrix.

The day may soon come when a dominatrix finds herself pleading her case before a judge who has visited her dungeon. The law can be a strange and wonderful thing. And few are more aware of that than a young New York City publisher who operates (barely) within the law and gets to say and depict all manner of outrageous things in his magazine. The mag is called *Vice*, and you can pick it up at fine, and not-so-fine, S&M joints everywhere.

The kudos just don't stop coming: "I love reading *Vice* magazine: it's ill" (Rhettmatic, Beat Junkies); "It's all right" (Johnny Rotten, ex-Sex Pistols singer); "Hard to believe that the hottest thing in New York right now comes from Montreal" (Kevin Bisch, *Details*); "Y'alls so goddamn sexy...gots my pecker so hard a cat couldn't scratch it" (Frank Kozik, Man's Ruin Records and top-shelf lowbrow artist); "How did you get this number?" (Spike Lee).

Pretty heady stuff. Suroosh Alvi, publisher and cofounder of *Vice*, drinks it all in at the mag's boho digs in New York City's funky Lower West Side. It wasn't so long ago that Alvi and his partners, Gavin McInnes and Shane Smith, were slackers living on welfare in Montreal. Now they've got an empire: *Vice* magazine, Vice Fashion, Vice Film, Vice Records, Vice T.V., and, of course, the Viceland.com Web site, which fuels the aforementioned.

Parallels may be drawn between the careers of Alvi and *Playboy* magnate Hugh Hefner — provided that you overlook the fact that Alvi is of Muslim stock, he's many decades younger than Hef, and he likes to fill his pages with guides to eating pussy and homages to dead sumo wrestlers. But, like Hef, Alvi has stuck to his guns. And sometimes when you refuse to bend to convention and play by the rules good things can happen — you might even prosper. Plenty of chutzpah has propelled Alvi and his partners to the lofty perch they now occupy in the Big Apple. Before *Vice*, it was just the *Voice*. To drum up a little publicity, the boys spread a rumor that the *Village Voice* was threatening to sue them over their name. The big ploy worked: the trio of Montreal upstarts received international coverage and a boost in circulation due to a bald-faced lie.

Almost as audacious was one particular tall tale propagated by Shane Smith. He revealed to a newspaper that the fabulously wealthy Richard Szalwinski, founder of the hugely successful software company SoftImage and owner of both the special-effects firm Discreet Logic and multimedia company Behaviour, was seeking to invest in *Vice*. Yet the *Vice* boys, who were having trouble keeping their mag afloat, had never even spoken to Szalwinski. Astonishingly, Szalwinski swallowed the bait. The boys, who hadn't a clue what their enterprise was worth, valued the biz at four million dollars and sold Szalwinski a twenty-five percent share for a cool million. There was a proviso, though. Szalwinski, who, unbeknownst to the boys, had always been hot on the mag, insisted that *Vice* move from Montreal to New York; become part of Szalwinski's mother ship, Normalnet; go international; and go public. So, in 1999, *Vice* pulled up stakes and relocated to New York. Circulation has since risen to nearly one hundred thousand copies, ten times a year. When the deal was finalized, Normalnet owned *Vice*; and Alvi, McInnes, and Smith, in turn, owned 7.5 percent of Normalnet, which encompasses close to twenty companies.

"*Vice* is the penultimate source for depraved urban culture," says Alvi with pride over a latte he's just made at the company's onsite coffee bar. "*Vice* is the future." Yet what began as a raunchy lifestyle mag that was embraced by the disenfranchised and disaffected between the ages of eighteen and twenty-nine, is now a raunchy lifestyle mag that is embraced by the mainstream (possibly even Spike Lee). Sex has a lot to do with that. "We were never afraid to talk about sex in print the way we would talk about it among our friends," Alvi notes. Which is to say, in the most graphic, outrageous terms possible.

Whereas the mainstream skin mags tend to dwell on sex from the male perspective, *Vice* is an equal-opportunity pervert, offering women lots of chances to get in on the action. One of the mag's most popular features is "Skinema," a collection of porno reviews from a female point of view. *Vice* has also been acclaimed for its guides to performing cunnilingus and fellatio. The former guide begins with this proclamation: "Men suck at eating pussy." It then goes on to describe techniques such as "parting the Red Seas" and to offer advice nuggets such as "don't say hi to dry." And where else would you find a tale of intimacy like "Lost in Uranus?" As the title implies, this piece is the confession of a woman who somehow wound up with an eight-inch dildo lost in her butt. Doctors feared that they might have to operate, but then good fortune intervened and the dildo just dropped out. Talk about groundbreaking sex coverage. Also, *Vice* achieved infamy of sorts with "Hump Day in Havana," a report on prostitution in Cuba. A similar no-holds-barred perspective was served up in "Pimping in America." And only *Vice* would venture to do a fashion spread featuring hookers that included their agency's numbers.

Hef contends that his magazine *Playboy* is about far more than sex, and Alvi says the same of his own publication. He breaks the *Vice* format down into six components, most of which would never find their way into *Playboy*: stupid content; smart content; sex; beats; guitars; and fashion. By stupid, Alvi means really stupid. Like taking pictures of feces filled with corn remnants or progressive shots of the Vice Gross Jar, a deteriorating amalgam of chicken parts, shit, and cigarette butts. Smart, however, would be a sobering look at surviving prison or an exposé of Eastern European serial killers. "What makes us unique on all subjects, including sex, is a different perspective than anyone else," Alvi maintains. "Other magazines have tried to duplicate us, but to no avail. We are the only free international magazine that deals this candidly with urban culture — and with fifty percent ads." Alvi attributes the attitude he and his partners share to their Montreal roots. "There's a quirky kind of openness in Montreal that you don't find anywhere else in the world. There is a hunger, much of which comes from a lack of money, that is contagious to readers."

Alvi took a circuitous route to journalism. He graduated with a philosophy degree from McGill University. He then worked as a rep for a music company in Minneapolis before heading to Slovakia to teach English for a year. But it was living on welfare that finally drove him and his cofounders to *Vice*. Some fear that since the stakes have risen so high the *Vice* boys might be tempted to sell out. Alvi dismisses the notion, saying, "We're not changing content one iota. This is more about cashing in than selling out." Nor does Alvi have difficulty reconciling

Vice with his Muslim roots: "I have my own spiritual beliefs and follow the religion in my own way."

Lately, Alvi has been communing with people he would never have had access to a few short years ago. One such individual is Patrick Gavin, Normalnet's senior vice president and chief financial officer. Gavin hails from a background to which Alvi can relate: he used to be a CFO and CEO at *Penthouse*; and he's bullish on *Vice*. "As long as it keeps changing with the times and speaks to its demographic," he says, "there is no stopping the magazine's potential. In the early days, *Penthouse* as a brand appealed to a lot of people and pushed the envelope, but then it became more a labor of love than a business for [founder and publisher] Bob Guccione. This is a tough business. Sex magazines start up every year, but there is a limited market. Those that succeed — like *Playboy* — distinguish themselves with editorials and mainstream ads." *Vice*, in Gavin's view, is a *Playboy/Penthouse* for another generation. "It's about lifestyle and it's niche oriented. There are lots of untapped pockets around the world which would be well served by *Vice*." Gavin hopes to spread the word through the Website as well as Vice fashions, films, and T.V. "*Vice* is not just a magazine. It's a multichannel approach to tapping into a market, using everything from print to clothing."

And this just in: the slacker kids have pulled off another coup. They've taken control of their empire (although Normalnet's Szalwinski remains a minor shareholder), and they've vacated the Normalnet space to set up shop in larger quarters in Brooklyn. And, while we're at it, this just in, too: rapper Beans of the Anti-Pop Consortium has this to say about Alvi, McInnes, and Smith's baby: "*Vice* is the most vulgar, loveable magazine with the most insane people behind it. How can you not love a magazine that gives points on eating out a girl?" Indeed. But insane? Insane like foxes, maybe.

Insanity runs rampant in the Big Apple, says the wee fellow sitting next to me, just in case I had any doubts. He also tells me that they call him the Rodent. Fine — I have no reason to disbelieve that he would be so dubbed. After all, it's a little before noon and we're the only patrons holding down stools in a ramshackle West Side bar at the epicenter of Manhattan's rough-and-tumble garment district. "But don't get the wrong impression about this Rodent business," my companion quickly adds. Apparently, it's a term of endearment. And envy. The Rodent, you see, can extricate himself from the sort of predicament that would bring the rest of us to our knees. No matter how dire the circumstances, no matter how far removed he is from his home base, the Rodent somehow manages to claw his way out and save his soul.

Speaking of soul. Actually, Seoul. Over a couple of triple martinis, the Rodent recalls what is perhaps his hairiest adventure to date. As an importer of swimsuits from the Orient and the Far East, he often facilitates his transactions by bringing his North American buyers — who work for a range of high-end department stores — along with him on overseas trips. This saves the Rodent a lot of legwork. But what these buyers are invariably focused on is not the prospect of meeting their suppliers in person. What excites them is the opportunity to dabble in the local culture and partake of some exotic delights. "Nookie," says the Rodent, just in case I failed to grasp his concept of exotica.

So, the Rodent and a buyer, let's call him Bob, find themselves holed up in some high-rent Seoul hotel in the dead of winter. Bob is delighted at whatever swimsuit arrangements the Rodent has made with the suppliers, but now Bob wants to get boffed. The Rodent dutifully calls a local escort service. Shortly thereafter, several women visit the Rodent's hotel room. Bob has a difficult choice to make. "Take one. Take two. It's up to you," the Rodent says obligingly. He is nothing if not magnanimous. The agent for the women makes only one stipulation. He insists to the Rodent that Bob take a shower before the frolicking begins. The Koreans are strong on cleanliness. They are also strong.

Bob takes the mandatory shower with the woman he has finally selected, but he can't contain his euphoria in the shower. This is a no-no. Patience is also a virtue in Korea. Meanwhile, the Rodent, believing everything to be under control, relaxes in the living room, puffing away on one of his beloved Churchill stogies. He has opened the window wide in order to avoid activating the smoke detector. The room is on the eighth floor, overlooking the hotel driveway. This seemingly inconsequential detail will come into play shortly, the Rodent informs me.

When Bob's woman enters the room wrapped in a towel, clearly upset about something, the Rodent is surprised. Bob has been bad, the lady charges. "Like many Koreans," recounts Bob, "she is very physical. She gives me a push to show her displeasure with Bob. But as she does so, I trip on the coffee table in the living room and then proceed to fly out the open window." The Rodent is not a very large person, the window has no screen, and it's eight floors up. Under normal circumstances, all of this would have resulted in tragedy, but by the grace of a higher power — one clearly oblivious to the Rodent's ways — the Rodent's free fall is broken by a flagpole a floor below.

"It's freezing out," the Rodent tells me. "I'm dangling for dear life on a flagpole in my bathrobe. I can't reach the room adjacent to the flagpole. So I sit on the pole like a putz, smoking my cigar, which I somehow managed to hold on to throughout the ordeal. Meanwhile, hotel guests are coming up the driveway and see me dangling there. They think I'm about to commit suicide. And inside the hotel, the hooker is running up and down the halls, absolutely hysterical. She thinks she's killed me and is considering suicide herself. Security guards are running all over the hotel, trying to figure out which room I fell out of and what to do. They call the Seoul fire and police departments. They arrive shortly with hooks and ladders and trampolines. And they start screaming in Korean and English, 'Please don't jump. Life can't be that bad. Let's talk.' And then the hooker comes to the window ready to jump, until she spots me on the pole and starts screaming even louder. And Bob the buyer, unaware of everything that has happened, is plain pissed off because he can't score with the woman."

The fire department was eventually able to hook the Rodent off the pole and carry him to safety. And everyone lived happily ever after — more or less. The Rodent tells me that he learned an important life lesson from all this. "About faith?" I ask meekly. The Rodent flashes me a most puzzled look. "Nah," he barks: "Keep the window shut while you're smoking a cigar."

The Rodent slips off his stool, narrowly avoids landing face down on the floor, and then splits. I am mystified. The bartender is not. He's a New Yorker. But then this bartender, as bartenders are wont to do when the joint is nearly empty, strikes up a conversation. He asks me what I'm doing in these parts. When I tell him, he seems mildly interested, but no more than that — from where he stands and pours, he's heard all manner of tales, and some are even true. "If you want my opinion . . . and I might add that it's free," he says. "Okay," I say. "Shoot." "Well," he continues, "you know where we are now?" Wild guess — "New York?" To that, the bartender replies "Yeah, yeah, smart guy." He just might be related to Mistress Otter. "Well, smart guy, before it was New York, it was . . . New Amsterdam." I counter, "And your point would be?" Then I'm told, "Well, smart guy, New York is a pretty raunchy city. So the way I see it, if this town was named after Amsterdam, then the real Amsterdam must be some kind of raunchy place, right?"

Right. Only from the mouths of babes and bartenders does this kind of logic get dispensed. Free of charge, too. Just as well, since my ensuing plane ride to old Amsterdam sure isn't.

Chapter 4

BIKES, DIKES, AND BANANAS?

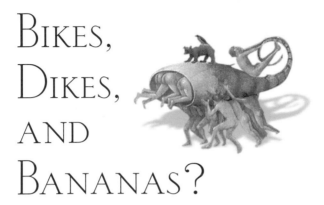

Onto the overhead television screen in Amsterdam's cozy Bar Bizonder flashes an attractive Russian T.V.-news anchor. She's delivering a report on a rousing speech Bill Clinton has just given to high-school students in the American heartland. The anchor then segues into a story about elections in Iran and follows it up with another about an upsurge on the Nasdaq exchange. Oh yes, and the whole time this poker-faced anchor is reading the news, she is delicately peeling off her clothing, piece by piece, without missing a beat. By the end of the newscast, she's buck naked.

The bar's predominantly Dutch clientele pay little attention to the broadcast. No cackles. No giggles. No moral outrage. Hey, what did you expect?

Welcome to Amsterdam, where it takes a whole lot more than a stripping Russkie news anchor to give locals pause as they quaff their mind-altering Jenever potions and brew-chasers. Amsterdam is a city of (at last count) 1,268,908 inhabitants, 145 nationalities, 400,000 nondesigner bicycles you couldn't foist at gunpoint on any North American hipster, 220,000 trees, 600,000 tulips, 1,281 bridges, 165 canals, 2,500 houseboats, 206 Van Goghs, 22 Rembrandts, 8 barrel organs, a mere 6 windmills, 1 royal palace, and 1 mother of a red light district that is bigger than the downtown sector of most any major metropolis on this planet. To say that Amsterdam is one of the most permissive cities on this planet is to drastically understate. This is a town pretty much without taboos. Virtually anything goes on the sex and soft-drug front. What is left to the imaginations of this town's burghers . . . you don't want to know. Short of lighting your spliff for you and handing you a prophylactic, Amsterdam city fathers and mothers couldn't be more accommodating to locals and tourists alike. Not only do they relish their vices, but they also advertise them.

Actually, the only thing left to the imagination in this town is: How much is that hooker in the window? According to Nelléy, a grandmotherly type wearing the sort of loungewear you never want to see your own grandma sporting the price, based on time and services rendered, is negotiable. Nelléy, by the bye, is neither a harlot nor a Keynesian economist. Rather, she toils at Absolute Danny, Amsterdam's most acclaimed emporium of erotica, which sits smack in the middle of the red light district. Despite the name, Danny is no dude. Indeed, Danny Linden is so proud of her torso that she and her mammoth naked mammaries, adorned with leathers and chains, are showcased in the shop's brochures. Nelléy is Danny's sixtysomething mom, and she couldn't be more proud of her kid. "We Dutch are not hypocrites," Nelléy opines. "We are proud of our openness towards sex. We are proud of our bodies. We are less proud, though, about our openness concerning our emotions. Hopefully, we will come around there, too."

Nelléy takes deep pride in displaying the wares of this upscale, dimly lit boutique. "It's all about class," she says. "There is nothing vulgar here — other than perhaps the thoughts of some who visit." Gosh, even the handcuffs come lined with some furlike substance — to avoid chafing, I'm told. In addition to hawking rubber corsets and racy videos and rocking devices that could register on the Richter scale, Danny is also an artist; her decidedly erotic abstracts are scattered throughout the store. But Danny herself is nowhere to be found on this day. She's vacationing in Thailand, another porn mecca. Not that she would have much to learn there — she's gone primarily to paint. Nelléy says that Danny will likely be back in a few weeks for her favorite fetish night, The Clinic, for which participants show up equipped with medical paraphernalia, fake plasma, and precious little clothing, to pay tribute to nurses, but not necessarily those of the Florence Nightingale ilk. Nelléy herself isn't sure whether she'll attend. Her hubby is less wild about medical-themed discos set in dungeons than she is, but she urges others to go, declaring that the champagne bar with the go-go nurses is a blast of epic proportions. "Just remember, though," she cautions, "the dress-code is strict." "Black tie for gents, you mean?" Nelléy gives me such a look. "No, no! You must come in rubber or leather or plastic. Or, if you wish, in a crossdress nurse's uniform. This way, the other participants won't feel so uncomfortable." Uh-huh.

A young German couple stroll into the store. Nelléy tries to interest the woman in a red rubber corset. "It never goes out of fashion, you know," she says in that sweet, grandmotherly voice of hers. "And how about a purple corset for your man?" The fella is a little mystified, especially by the zipper on the lower portion of the purple corset. "Oh, that's the penis pouch," Nelléy cheerfully explains. The couple confer seriously about purchasing the merch.

A matronly British lady and her patronly husband saunter into the store. In an eerie, Maggie Thatcher-like tone, the lady requests to see the famed Tarzan vibrator. "We heard all about it on the Internet," she tells Nelléy. "Apparently, it can give enormous pleasure in many different ways, soft and hard," her significant other chimes in. Nelléy smiles, nods, and produces the Tarzan, which looks formidable enough to take on a herd of elephants, let alone a middle-aged couple from Leeds.

Meanwhile, the young Germans are debating whether one of them would look better in a nurse's bra emblazoned with a smart red cross or the ever-popular spider bra — which appears somewhat impractical, as it offers no visible means of support. But I digress. As always, Nelléy has the appropriate solution: "Well, if you plan on attending our Clinic fetish night, the nurse's bra is a must. But if it's just for a little spark in the bedroom, then by all means go for the spider bra." At this point, the British matron trumpets, "Har-rold! Don't you think I'd look smashing in a spider?" To which the flummoxed Harold wisely replies, "Yes, dear."

Stationed at the cash register, observing all of this activity, is Diana, another Absolute Danny employee. Diana used to crack a whip for a living. She was a successful dominatrix at a dungeon in The Hague. Sadly, an accident that cost her an eye forced Diana out of that field; she maintains that it was just too hard to crack a whip at one client and keep watch over another with just one eye. So you're thinking that Diana's accident involved an errant lash, but you're wrong. "In ten years working with a whip in a dungeon, I never had any accidents," she says. In fact, Diana lost her eye while trying to help a young man she saw writhing in pain on a sidewalk. Unfortunately, the guy was in a crazed stupor and he unloaded on the Good Samaritan Diana with a flurry of punches to the eye, inflicting such damage that her doctors had little choice but to remove the eye and replace it with a (perfectly matched) artificial one.

Diana is remarkably philosophic about the ordeal, although she does miss the dungeon. "It was more erotic than sexual," she says. "It was actually quite social and I met some fine people." She is referring to the military and United Nations types from around the world who were stationed in The Hague. "Every client I had left with a smile. It was like my personal guarantee." Like many in the biz, Diana believes that she was performing an important service for her predominantly married clientele. "It was simply a case of men going to another store when their wives wouldn't perform at their store. But there was no love involved. Just an exchange of friendship — and about a thousand guilders a night for me."

Although close to 50, Diana looks fifteen years younger. She talks like a therapist, not a tramp. "One of my favorite clients was a high-ranking Dutch officer who served with United Nations peacekeeping forces in Bosnia. He was my slave, and he loved it. He even tried to send fellow officers to visit me as a way of balancing them out, too. After giving orders to others all day in warlike situations, it was a relief for him to take orders instead." Even if that meant panting like a rottweiler and crawling naked on all fours around Diana's makeshift dungeon.

But no time for reminiscing. An earnest Dutch housewife walks into the store and asks for info about the Pocket Rocket. This gizmo turns out to be a hot property — a minivibrator that can provide relief almost anywhere at a moment's notice. "Satisfaction is guaranteed," Diana reassures the woman. "Provided, of course, that you remember to keep fresh batteries handy." The ladies then embark on a lengthy discussion concerning the potency of various battery brands. The Germans and the Brits join in. Naturally, Nelléy has an opinion as well: "The bunny. Always the bunny brand."

I need some air, so off I scamper. I continue my exploration of this town where almost every enterprise is provocatively named and rich in innuendo. This brings me to the Big Bananas Night Shop. It brings a lot of other tourists here, too. Thys Overgoor, the store's manager, spends most of his days giggling. "People come in and get the wrong impression," he says. "They suspect something strange is going on — but, really, all we do is sell fruit here, including many bananas. Really." The confusion is understandable. One of the hottest spots in Amsterdam is the Bananenbar, where naked acrobatic bartending ladies perform astonishing feats with the banana fruit while mixing libations for their grateful customers. So Thys Overgoor kindly directs his confused tourists to Bananenbar and occasionally sells them a few bananas, as well. "The important thing is that bananas are good for you, no matter how you use them," says Mona, a youthful Big Bananas clerk. "All the same, people get the wrong impression about this store in general, and bananas in particular."

Irony abounds in Amsterdam. The Garlic Queen, for example, is a resto that specializes in garlicky dishes and that is decorated with pictures of genuine monarchs who reign over fiefdoms, such as the fair Beatrix of the Netherlands and England's Elizabeth. The Real Live Fucking Show, located on another quaint, canal-lined street in the red light district, is, in fact, a cabaret featuring real live fucking. Not that the rowdy, beer-swilling English soccer fans who've filled the place on this brisk afternoon need any more enticement than real beer.

They hoot and holler as a striking, scantily clad woman in a blonde wig appears on the stage and levitates a horizontal man in a cape a few feet off the floor. "Ya gonna fuck now, or what, honey?" screeches one scholar from the cheap seats. "'Ave some sex now, will ya darlin'?" his pal bellows. The woman seems oblivious. She turns her attention to another group of spectators who are showing much more restraint. "Hello, Japan," she coos, as the caped man strokes her breasts. "And remember, gentlemen, no pictures," she adds. She then proceeds to levitate another part of her partner's anatomy in the time-honored oral tradition. A few moments later, the man in the cape is shtupping her while she chats up the Japanese delegation. "Your glasses are getting all steamed up," she tells one of the Japanese gents. Looking past him, she asks a guy sitting in the row behind where he's from. "New York," the guy says. "You're kidding," she replies. "I have a friend in New York. Maybe you know him. His name is Peter." The man acknowledges that he knows a Peter.

I don't know if the Dutch hand out awards to their porno performers, but darn — you really have to admire the man in the cape. He is able to keep humping while his lady makes small talk and the soccer rowdies belch and the Japanese businessmen take illicit snapshots — with a flash, no less.

It's intermission time. The Real Live Fucking Show's cordial bartender, Bob, tells me that the club draws customers from Russia, the United States, Germany, Japan, and France. "But, without question, the British are the worst," he states. "And that's *before* they've loaded up on beer." Yet, while the management tolerates the Brits and even those customers who come in with their dogs, the club's no-smoking policy is strictly enforced, to the point where a performance will be halted if an offending cigarette isn't extinguished. So imagine my surprise when the next attraction takes to the stage with a lit stogie. But this babe is soon blowing smoke in a way one would never have thought possible. Even the babbling Brits are taken aback and silenced. "What muscles," one soccer fans finally murmurs, marveling at the young lady's ability to re-light her cigar utilizing only the muscles of her astonishing vaginal tract. She pulls the burning stogie from her lower front orifice, places it in her mouth, and takes a few puffs. "Ew, that's bloody disgusting!" The Brits have found their tongues. "What are you, love?" one of them shouts. "Another Monica Lew-insky?" His friends titter.

A dog barks at the loudmouth Brit. The Brit barks back. Pandemonium breaks out as another caped performer, Zorro, struggles to maintain his concentration. He's performing push-ups on his lovely partner. Just when it seems like we're in store for a full-fledged soccer riot, the biggest bouncer I've ever seen in my life lumbers down the aisle towards the soccer fans, and suddenly they're as quiet as choir boys. "'E's a bloody good actor," one of the boys tells the impassive bouncer. "Imagine that — to roger his mate and still keep smiling like that. A bloody good actor, I tell you."

The show has ended. The bouncer gets up on the stage: "Get the fuck out of here! Now!" We think he's kidding. But who wants to quibble with a seven-foot, three-hundred-pound gargantuan who isn't smiling? I go to speak with Paul, the club's manager, who fills me in on customer relations. Of the British clientele, he says, "They come down here to get drunk and yell with their friends. Then they go home and don't even remember having come to Amsterdam for the weekend. But we rarely have fights here." That, of course, has everything to do with the presence of the world's biggest bouncer. His name turns out to be Winand. He tells me, "Sometimes the English don't always leave as fast as I tell them, so I help move them out a bit and they get out real fast." Winand is my new best friend. "Sometimes, a foolish person who is drunk will challenge me to a fight," he continues. "But I tell them I've never lost a fight in my life, and I probably never will, unless Mike Tyson ever shows up here." Paul interjects, "And even then, I'd bet on Winand." Winand protests, "But I'm a peaceful lad!" Whatever you say, Winand.

Night has fallen on Amsterdam. I know this for a fact, because tiny red lights come on in thousands of tiny cubicles — each of which boasts a seminude woman and a bed — all over the city's red light district. Hmm. Everything goes in the red light district. Handcuff-packing men and women in identical leather outfits skip through the streets looking like they're auditioning to be Village People cops. Ooops, they *are* cops. Sorry, officers. And The Finger in the Dyke? No, it's not what you're thinking. It's a restaurant that serves mussels.

Not time to chow down just yet. Time for some culture, a Walking Tour of Dark Amsterdam. It was the brochure that sold me: "A tour through 'Dark' Amsterdam can be rather illuminating because of the visit to the famous Red Light District. The excursion starts at a Prostitute Information Center, where we will offer you a drink." Damned civilized, those Dutch. At the meeting point, I discover that my fellow walkers look more like a church group than a gang of sleazoid voyeurs. I'm talking blue-haired British ladies and their tweed-attired, stiff-upper-lipped husbands; bespectacled American computer nerds; and, of course, the ubiquitous Japanese. Our tour guide is the dour Wouter, who is probably the last guy on the planet you'd pick to lead a walk on the wild side. Wouter is an idealist and, quite probably, a socialist. Which is fine. He's also virtually humorless.

Which is less fine. "Through the ages, we have had a tradition of tolerance in Amsterdam," Wouter announces as our adventure begins. "We even took in Protestants who were kicked out of France. And you're probably wondering about our name." Now that you mention it, Wouter, no. Wouter goes on to explain anyway: "There was a dam in the Amstel River. Hence, Amsterdam." Ah.

"But what about the hookers, Wouter?" one British gent inquires. "Yes, yes. I'll get to that," answers the stern-faced guide, "but first stop, a condom shop. Condoms are important and safe. They can prevent disease." Thank you, Wouter. Condoms can also be fun, judging by those we see arrayed before us — there's Rudolph the Red-Nosed Reindeer, the Statue of Liberty, Homer Simpson . . . "Oh, I quite fancy that one," a giddy, British blue hair says to her husband. "He looks a little like you, don't you think?" Hubby is unamused. The condom in question is the Homer Simpson special.

No time to dawdle. Wouter has launched into a new spiel, about logs cracking in the water in the red light district. Methinks Wouter is making metaphors. "This area is unlike all the rest in the city," he pronounces. "What was your first clue, Wouter? The lingerie-clad twins over there in the window doing stretching exercises for the pedestrians?" "No, no, no!" he scolds me. "I'm talking about the coffee shops." In all fairness to Wouter, he ain't talking Starbucks. Coffee shops have a far different significance in this town. Clients don't go for the Moka Java, they go for the marijuana. Coffee-shop proprietors are permitted to sell five grams of pot to each customer and may keep more than five hundred grams on the premises. Swell, right? Wouter shakes his head. "While it is permitted to sell the stuff, the coffee-shop owner cannot legally buy the marijuana from anyone. This is a dilemma, no?"

So those fun-loving Dutch have a few free-market glitches to work out. On the subject of the free market, a hooker takes exception to the fact that Wouter has decided to deliver his sermon on the mount directly in front of her window, thus blocking the view of prospective clients. She starts banging against the tiny window with a hairbrush, but Wouter is oblivious. It takes one of the British blue hairs to bring the situation to his attention, but he's more intent on pointing out The Bulldog, the region's first coffee house, established circa 1968 in a marijuana haze.

Wouter next leads us down the narrowest alley in the world — it's about a yard wide. On either side, hookers gaze out from the windows of their tiny rooms. Wouter seizes this opportunity to tell us that when the curtains are drawn, it's a good bet that people are engaged in sex therein. Thanks, Wouter.

By a quirk of fate, the oldest church in Amsterdam is located in the part of the city where the world's oldest profession is practiced. More food for thought, Wouter suggests. "And, for your information, ladies and gentlemen," he continues, "the red lights indicate a room belonging to a hooker, while the white lights indicate homes of just regular people." Wouter is beginning to insult the intelligence of many in our group. "Blimey, does he think we were born yesterday?" one blue hair asks her tweedy mate.

Now it's time for the much-promised visit to the Prostitute Information Center and that free drink. A cheerful woman named Miriam took on the job of running this establishment after paying dues on the street. "I became a prostitute because I was a really lousy waitress," she confides. The Brits giggle. The place is a drop-in center for the area's working girls. And what kind of information are they seeking? Miriam says that what they want to know about most is, of all things, taxes. When prostitution was legalized, Dutch tax collectors decreed that the red light ladies contribute to the nation's coffers. "The girls want to pay these taxes, too, but they just never know how much and how often," Miriam explains. So Miriam has become the H&R Block of the red light district. "We also get customers dropping by, asking all sorts of questions," she says, "but I have to be delicate and tell them we're not shrinks, just hookers here." The center sells condoms, as well, and the proceeds go to the hooker tax fund. Plus, the center features a sample hooker room — equipped with a bed and a window — for the benefit of the imaginatively challenged.

Miriam explains the rules of the game. A hooker pays up to seventy-five dollars to rent a room for an eight-hour shift. Apart from the spartan bed, the room is furnished with an alarm and a video camera — which could prove to be very alarming to a customer. According to Miriam, though, videos are held for only twenty-four hours and then taped over; it's almost unheard-of for anyone to use a video for blackmail purposes.

All that a prostitute needs to practice her trade legally in the Netherlands is a passport proving that she is over eighteen years old and a citizen of a European Union country. "I know that many feel sorry for these women, because people pass by and look at them like they're monkeys in a zoo," comments Miriam. "Sure, there are some unfortunate women in this business. But, believe me, most are happy. They're making very good money. They work under sanitary conditions and they feel quite secure. They also feel like they're providing an important social service for the community." While the government offers prostitutes free health checks — authorities recommend a physical every three months — they aren't compulsory. The hookers themselves inspect their clients. Says Miriam, a client may find himself being given "a severe wash of the genital area with the strongest soap money can buy." Condoms are, of course, mandatory.

Miriam notes that clients have little time to forge relationships with the girls, because a session rarely lasts longer than ten minutes. "The man might forget the time, but the woman never does," she adds. Occasionally, a ringing alarm may be heard in the red light district, but, as Miriam explains, "it's almost always because the customer is haggling over the time. Violence here is extremely rare."

According to Wouter, Amsterdam's red light district has been around for seven hundred years. And according to Miriam, the girls are proud to be upholders of the tradition. "In a perfect world, everyone would have a fairy-tale romance and great sex with their mates," she reflects. "But that is the stuff of fantasy. That's why prostitution is a fact of life." Yet another grand tradition prevails in this city: women never pay for sex. "That's why we have five hundred unemployed gigolos in Amsterdam," Miriam smiles.

When Miriam decided to leave the trade a number of years back, it wasn't because she found the work demeaning or unpleasant. Au contraire — she quite enjoyed it. "It wasn't the work," she says. "I was making a really good living, just like someone with a university degree might make. No, it was more because I was living a lie, a double life. I came from a middle-class family and I was worried about hurting my parents if they found out what I was doing. So I lied, but I felt like such a hypocrite." The experience didn't sour her on men, either. "Men are like Germans. We don't like 'em, but we need 'em." She's joking, I think.

Back on the street, one of the blue hairs suddenly shrieks, "Will ya look at the size of those jugs!" She scares the bejesus out of her husband and nearly everyone else within earshot. The lady does, however, have some justification for her outburst. We've just passed a window occupied by a woman whose anatomy defies both gravity and current means of measurement. Wouter, in a rare moment of levity, asks us if we would like to join him in prayer at Our Lord in the Attic, yet another neighborhood church. This one, as its name implies, is housed on a top floor, and us would-be worshippers are reluctant to climb all those stairs. "Anyway, God has yet to be found in this attic," Wouter remarks.

And God knows what to make of a place called The Bingo House. Bingo in the red light district? It's a place where hookers go to play bingo in their off hours, silly. In fact, one hooker we encounter on her way into The Bingo House maintains that bingo is the only thing that brings her to the red light district these days. "It's become too touristy," she says. "It scares off real customers. So we've moved to another area." She doesn't want to tell us where, fearing that if she does Wouter will show up with one of his walking tours.

Not even the blue hairs blink an eye as we pass a flowing fountain in the shape of a gi-normous penis. After an hour on the street, nothing shocks us any longer. Even Wouter seems bored and he starts drawing our attention to architectural details that have squat to do with sex. "Look how delightfully the ceilings are painted," he intones. "And look at those hooks on the top of the buildings." This isn't code for hookers at work. Rather, because so many of these historic buildings have very narrow entrances, tight staircases, and no elevators, a system was devised hundreds of years ago to hoist furniture with a rope affixed to a hook. Today, movers still use the contraption, but they have to figure out a way to unhinge a building's huge front windows before they can get the furniture inside. "Now I've really learned something," a blue hair tells Wouter. He is pleased. Some of us, though, are baffled.

If it's Sunday, it must be family day at Amsterdam's Sex Museum. The brochure proclaims that this is the only sex museum in Europe — unless, of course, you count The Erotic Museum, located only a few blocks away from this establishment in the red light district. It's ten in the morning, and already the place is filled, not with leering pervs, but with decent-looking folk: Japanese couples, a group of British high school girls, and — surprise — a number of real-live Dutch families in pursuit of culture. Now, whether or not the whip-toting male mannequin with the nipple clamps and leather underwear at the museum's entrance constitutes culture is open to debate. The museum is a hodgepodge of porn art and kinky pop-culture artifacts. On one wall, the erotic paintings of nineteenth-century Austrian artist Peter Fendi are showcased. And on another hangs the ever-popular lesbos-in-bondage homage. Fendi, as you are all doubtless aware, was a favorite of the those slap happy Hapsburgs; but we're not sure what their feelings were towards the babes in bondage.

The Sex Museum is cleverly, if not a little mischievously, designed. A steady chorus of "eeewww"s emanating from the British schoolgirls ahead indicates that something foul awaits the rest of us. Sure enough, while ascending the staircase, visitors are treated to an array of sculpted torsos, breasts, and at least one set of buttocks that is triggered by a motion detector to pass wind. Ah, those kooky Dutch are at it again.

The museum does what it can to provide insight into the world of telephone sex. Visitors are encouraged to pick up phones and listen to couples moaning and groaning in a dialect that is apparently meant to represent the language of love. Nearby is a fetching shot of a nude Swiss skier in the act of throwing caution and fear of frostbite to the winds. Then there is a display of erotic pipes — the smoking variety — and plates — the dinner variety. The dildo display is also unique, although the jury is out as to whether the creator of the whale-toothed sculpture actually had unorthodox sex in mind. Americans will be touched by the impressive sculpted monument to Marilyn Monroe. The museum's curators have gone so far as to display her standing on a subway vent, air blasting up her dress, just like in that famous scene from *The Seven Year Itch*. This is the most tame objet d'art to be found in the museum. Not far from it is a risqué arrangement of giant penis bronzes and colorful toilet-seat sketches.

History buffs will get a kick out of the vintage fifties porno oeuvres of the famed Candy Barr, who is showcased in the buff. "It's interesting how so little has changed in the technique of sex over the years," one astute visitor comments to his wife. "No matter the technology of today, the equipment remains the same." "Quite," utters the wife.

Warning: think twice before you sit on those chairs next to the penis bronzes. In response to the slightest movement, they generate unexpected vibrations that will jar the squeamish and amuse the silly no end. And watch out for that grotesque big breasted mama sculpture that not only moves but actually lurches out at stunned visitors. And don't be fooled by the multi-penis-shaped ashtray — smoking is absolutely verboten at The Sex Museum. Fornicate where and with whom you will in this town, but smoke in a restricted area, and you will be executed, just like Mata Hari. By the bye, a tribute to the Dutch-born spy and courtesan — who was executed without benefit of blindfold by a firing squad — is rather moving. So, too, for different reasons, is the tummy-turning display of humans having sex with animals over the ages. I swear I will never be able to look a horse or a snake square in the eye again. And what would any such museum be without an exhibit of erotic pastry? Decorative cakes — like the one with "Happy Breast Day" inscribed on it — prove that the vagina and the penis have their place in the world of pastry making. It's a tasteful way to end a tour of the museum.

"Answer me this," a pensive, middle-aged Scottish fellow says to his wife as they prepare to leave. "I'm surrounded by startling sexual images, so how come I'm not horny?" His wife, staring blankly at a piece called Dirty Dicks, replies, "Frankly, I've been more aroused by a visit to the butcher's shop." A most valid point. Dare we say we've uncovered the Dutch Paradox? The Dutch can get as down and dirty as they like, they can display all manner of alleged erotica, but it's about as much of a turn-on as catching Mickey Mouse without his skivvies.

Next, I trek over to the nearby Erotic Museum for a little comparison shopping. This may have been a mistake. As soon as I enter, I'm treated to a graphic photo depicting venereal disease in some sorry fellow's testicles. I feel like hurling my herring. On the floors above, yet more period porno is flashed on myriad screens. If porno playing cards crank your knob, you'll be in heaven when you come to an adjacent display. Erotic might not be the word that pops up into the minds of some visitors as they scope late Beatle John Lennon's drawings of his wife, Yoko Ono. The animated porno take on Snow White and the Seven Dwarfs comes as a breath of fresh air after Yoko. Less subtle is the S&M torture chamber on the top floor, replete with a bound lady mannequin pissing over visitors' heads. Fortunately, a sheet of plexiglass has been installed to keep our hair dry.

I do believe I've overdosed on raunch. So it's off to a coffee house for some much-needed substance abuse. My luck. I pick the only coffee house in all of Amsterdam that actually sells coffee and tea and not the mind-altering substances that Wouter mentioned. Over a cup of mint tea, I start perusing the personal ads of the Amsterdam daily newspaper *De Volks Krant*. It's immediately apparent that this is a futile exercise, largely because I don't understand Dutch. Offering a free cup of mint tea, I conscript the real-live Dutch person sitting at the next table to translate for me. I explain to the young man — whose name is Max — that I am looking for insights into the mating habits of real-live Dutch people, and I figure the personals are a capital place to begin. Max looks at me like I've just landed from some distant planet — which is something, considering that almost nothing fazes real-live Dutch people. Somewhat apprehensively, he starts to read: "Fifty-four-year-old man wants to fall in love again. He offers culture, biking, and walking. He seeks slender, blue-eyed, forty-year-old woman." Max yawns. "Sounds like a loser." Then he finds a dilly: "Older gentleman who never wears a tie but can sing beautifully wants to meet a woman, up to fifty, who can sing, who is tender and who has long hair, because long hair is the antenna of good intentions." Those kooky Dutch again. I spit up my mint tea. Max moves on: "Looking for a millionaire? Then go to another ad. I am not rich, I am fifty-three, slim, and employed. I want someone to escape with me from reality to an exotic country. A little money of your own would help."

Max tries to explain to me that his countrypeople aren't quite as romantic as foreigners might suspect. I suspect he's saying this because he'll be damned if he's going to translate another ad for me. He asks permission to leave. Before he goes, though, he is kind enough to toss a magazine called *The Amsterdam Times* my way. It's in English. "Go crazy," Max tells me.

Stop the presses. This headline leaps right out at me: "Brothel

Chain Plans Airport Outlet." The story that follows explains, "The Dutch brothel chain Yab Yum intends to open a branch at Amsterdam's Schipol Airport to cater to stressed passengers. Passengers will be treated to a luxury welcome with champagne and caviar and can opt for a relaxing massage, spokesman Theo Heuft explained. He said the Yab Yum Caviar Club would primarily target those in transit with time between planes or early arrivals looking to unwind after a stressful flight. Local authorities are believed to be receptive to the idea, but Yab Yum will have to wait until building work at the airport is completed and space in the departures area becomes available. Amsterdam Schipol Airport is reluctant to discuss the initiative and has no comment for the moment. Brothels are legal in the Netherlands since the Dutch Senate approved a change in the law in October, 1999."

So, exactly where in the departures lounge will the boinking take place? Inquiring minds want to know. I ask Max, who has returned to the table. He shakes his head, but he does pass on a news flash that he's just heard on the radio: Vibrators will soon be sold in Dutch drugstores. Max explains that this initiative has something to do with relieving stress without the added stress of having to go to a sex shop to cop a vibrator.

Maybe it's just me. But suddenly it occurs to me that even the sidewalk barricades on the streets of Amsterdam are shaped like penises. Max and I agree that penis-shaped sidewalk barricades probably brought on the decline of Roman civilization way back when. All the same, be careful what you touch while trolling the streets of Amsterdam.

"Paris thinks about it. London talks about it. Rome dreams about it. But Amsterdam has it." And we ain't talking Heineken here. This is the sales pitch for The Casa Rosso, which only sounds like the sort of romantic Italian eatery where candles burn softly in wax-encrusted Chianti bottles and checkered tablecloths rule. In fact, The Casa Rosso, as millions of contented visitors from around the world can attest, is the cream — and

I use that word carefully — of the Amsterdam porno scene. The oldest and most renowned erotic theater in town, it is situated in the heart of the red light district.

Time was, no trip to Amsterdam was complete without a tour of the Heineken brewery and all the beer you could guzzle. These days, The Casa Rosso is an obligatory stop on the itinerary of any tourist — not just the hormonally jangled. Like just about every other sex hotspot in Amsterdam, The Casa Rosso draws much of its clientele from the well-heeled strata of Europe, North America, and the Orient. They fill the theater's 160 luxury fauteuils for the invariably sold-out weekend evening performances. Cheap, it isn't — tickets are almost sixty dollars a pop. But ambiance is everything in erotica. Give 'em a seedy venue with soiled carpets that stink of spilled booze, and you will attract the trenchcoats and Brit soccer fans en masse. But give 'em a touch of class, and they'll be convinced that the hard-core sex acts they're paying to watch are high art. Indeed, the Casa Rosso experience has become so desirable to so many that the theater's management has set up a Web site, where the only viruses are of a technical nature.

Casa Rosso performers let their imaginations run rampant. This is not merely your basic lick-it-and-stick-it act. There's a little cloak-and-dagger activity, too. Witness the engaging young couple who have brought their James Bond routine to the Casa Rosso stage. Complemented by an upbeat soundtrack and sophisticated lighting, James, revolving around the stage on a circular bed, is able to rise to the occasion — literally — and save the world after many of his body parts are stimulated by an obliging female helper. Once his strength has been restored, James and his partner engage in what looks like a harmonious Jane Fonda workout.

The second act of the evening commences with a rousing rendition of "Hey, Big Spender." Two elderly Spanish women sitting in front of the theater are so taken with the tune that they start singing along, snapping their fingers, and tapping their feet. For a minute, you might think you're at New York's

Radio City Music Hall. But that illusion is quickly shattered when Latino Lolly takes the stage. This comedy performer is no Rockette. After shedding layers of feather boas, she gets down to business and pulls the world's longest string of beads out of her crotch. Astounding. There are sport utility vehicles on the market with less luggage capacity than Latino Lolly. And the Spanish ladies just keep on singing and tapping their toes — you could be excused for thinking you've landed in some Fellini flick.

When Latino Lolly exits, she is replaced by a young man and woman who copulate perfectly and very energetically to the beat of a disco tune. The audience applauds politely, much the way they would after a subdued staging of a Chekhov play. There are no catcalls. There is no cackling. There is simply a show of respect for the professionalism of a pair of hard-working artistes. Of course, this level of decorum could be attributed to the fact that there are no rowdy British soccer fans in the house. It's actually a pity that there aren't, because the next act, Vicky, the whip-snapping dominatrix, would have kept them all in line. Since there are no brutes about, Vicky is forced to select a more respectable Brit from the crowd. She brings him onstage, clamps a studded dog collar around his neck, attaches a leash to it, shoves a huge T-bone in her victim's mouth, and walks him around the stage. When necessary, she yanks the leash to quicken his pace. The gentleman's wife, sitting safely in the audience seems far more amused than he does, particularly when the dominatrix attaches a plastic penis to his head and invites him to plunge it into her privates. The kicker is that the plastic appendage is flaccid, and Mr. Penis-Head's efforts are doomed to fail — much to the delight of the roaring audience.

The show's producers clearly have an overripe sense of the absurd. Why else would they have a fellow dressed as Batman hump along to Bob Dylan's "Knockin' on Heaven's Door"? Then, back by popular demand, Vicky reappears. She has shed her whips and leathers for less menacing Calypso gear, all the better to perform "The Banana Boat Song." So, this being Amsterdam, just about everyone in the house is expecting Vicky to execute awesome feats with my once-favorite fruit. But no. Vicky does a straight and inspired Calypso dance routine. Then she invites three of the most rhythmically challenged men she can find to join her. They line up behind her onstage, as does a guy in a gorilla suit. It's all very wholesome until the guy in the gorilla suit undoes his fly and playfully nudges the fellow in front of him with his gargantuan pecker — which may or may not be real. The audience is in hysterics. To show that there are no hard feelings, so to speak, Vicky pulls the offending penis off the gorilla and demonstrates that it is only plastic. Everyone goes home happy, save for the gorilla's victim, who is being taunted mercilessly by his wife.

The bartenders and waiters who toil at these establishments tend to be among the most genial folk you'll meet in all of Amsterdam. "The idea is not to threaten the customers," Casa Rosso bartender Sergio tells me, "but to make them feel as relaxed as they might be at home." Provided, of course, your home is furnished with revolving beds, a Batman lookalike, and the voluptuous Miss Vicky. Adds Mike, a waiter: "Don't forget that half our customers are women. So we have to take a much more polite and compassionate approach than we would if there were only men. I really love my work. Sure, there's a lot of running around, but the customers, for the most part, are terrific. And our work is not nearly as demanding as it is for the performers."

Mike has a point. Batman and Bond must get it on six times a night with their respective partners. Hard enough for most mere mortals to perform six times a night, but to do so on a stage in front of hundreds of strangers has to be one of the most demanding jobs known to man. "They see it basically as just a job," continues Mike. "But it certainly helps that these performers are couples living together. They are in love and know each other intimately. But while some are up for the challenge, others just can't handle it." Mike confides that some do wilt like tired tulips under the pressure.

Sergio informs me that staff members never get sidetracked and start gawking at the onstage acrobatics when they should be serving booze. "The funny thing is that we look but we just don't see anything onstage any more. I don't spend my evenings in an overstimulated state. People in the audience come up to me after the show and say they've had a terrific time, but the show hasn't left them horny. Well, that's what it's all about — to entertain audiences but not to get them horny. This isn't really porno. It's entertainment that happens to have a sexual edge."

Nowhere else in the world, Mike assures me, could such activities be conducted with the same degree of civility. "There are no taboos in the Netherlands. That helps. People are so open and tolerant that nothing is considered sleazy. What other red light district in the world could families walk through and feel as relaxed as they do here? If you show that the act of sex is a thing of love and no big deal, people don't develop all these repressed attitudes and become strange. It's just another fact of life." Thank you, Dr. Joyce Brothers.

Don't know what Dr. Joyce would make of the Bananenbar, a peel's throw from The Casa Rosso. As blasé about sex as one begins to get in Amsterdam, a visit to the Bananenbar is still an arresting experience. As its name suggests, this is an environment where the banana is king. The first thing visitors notice upon entering is that the bartenders are sitting *on* the bar — on plush cushions, actually. And they aren't your Mikes or Sergios either. They are women, and they are naked, and they perform astonishing feats with bananas while they mix you a screwdriver, or whatever else you choose. The Bananenbar gives new meaning to the notion of the in-your-face bartender. Its staff members appear to have been recruited from the Barnum and Bailey Circus. They dance with bananas. They warm bananas. They jettison bananas from their nether regions. And they invite you, the visitor, to eat those very bananas as part of a balanced diet.

Inez, one of the establishment's supple bartenders, makes a confession to me: "Before I started work here, I really used to love bananas. Now I don't care if I ever see or eat one again." But I want to know why the Dutch are bananas about bananas. I am told in no uncertain terms: "Because the Banana Bar sounds a lot better than the Cucumber Bar." Thank you, Inez. Inez is remarkably relaxed. And for an excellent reason. She doesn't have to worry about getting hassled by customers. Her boyfriend, who has a chest like a beer barrel, is the Bananenbar's bouncer. "It's really only the English we have to worry about," she says. "They start drinking and don't stop, and they get a little bent." While Inez is talking, I see out of the corner of my eye that another bartender, T.P., has begun to nibble affectionately on a customer's neck. Ever so deftly, she pops a previously invisible banana from her crotch. It flies several feet through the air before another customer fields it and then devours it.

Inez is explaining to me that at Bananenbar four bartenders work in tandem, each demonstrating her own specialty. Inez herself is the banana queen; T.P. is a wiz with a vibrator; Lisa does various kinds of massage, often involving a banana; and Andrea is the wordsmith of the bunch, penning surprisingly legible postcards without using her hands. Andrea is also something of a magician: she's able to take tips from her customers and make them disappear into her various orifices.

Some British businessmen want Inez to get the show started. "Ever seen a banana dance?" she teases. "No," the gents respond in unison. And darned if Inez doesn't make her banana do the funkiest dance you could imagine. Then, after peeling that lively banana, she reinserts it in her privates, garnishes it with a little whipped cream, and invites each Brit to take a bite. They all do, albeit a little reluctantly. Sensing their discomfort, Inez asks if they'd like to take the last remaining bit of the banana home in a doggy bag. After Inez completes her shtick, I ask her why she puts a condom on the banana at the beginning of her act. She looks at me a little sternly. "Because you never know where it's been. You can't be too careful with your fruit, you know."

Lisa is busily spreading Nivea all over her upper body. She invites the Brits to massage her. "The beauty of this job," says Lisa, "apart from the tips, is that it's been very good for my skin." She's serious. On the receiving end of ten to fifteen such massages a night, Lisa has lovely skin.

Next, Andrea takes over, demonstrating her penmanship to the Brits. They are bowled over. With her writing instrument nearly hidden, Andrea is able to manipulate her pelvis in such a way that she can jot on a postcard: "Dear Arnold. Big Kisses. From Pussy." She gets a richly deserved standing ovation. In fact, we are all so enthralled with Andrea's antics that we fail to notice that a sizable group of patrons has just entered the bar. They're big and bearded, and they wear colorful jean jackets. Hells Angels New York. Hells Angels California. Hells Angels Connecticut. Hells Angels England.

A dozen international Hells Angels have moved in next to me at the bar. My life flashes before my eyes. I am suddenly stone cold sober. Help! Where is Winand when I need him? I've begun to have hot flashes, and Inez thinks this is hysterical. She thinks it's even more hysterical that I ask her to please retrieve my coat for me — it's hanging at the end of the bar where the Angels are stationed. She asks if I could possibly wait until she's finished making her banana split for the Angels. Sure, fine. Fortunately, the Angels are consumed with Inez and Andrea and T.P. and Lisa and their bananas; they pay no heed to the fellow slinking out of the bar, desperately trying to hold on to the contents of his bladder. "You've read too many newspapers and have watched too much television," Inez jests as I exit. Precisely.

I reckon that the time has come to leave swinging Amsterdam. I decide to hightail it to Paris, city of romance and light and philosophers and swell bistros and octogenarian hookers.

Chapter 5

MOULIN ROUGED

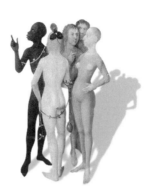

PARIS

Okay, so what gives? The road signs all say Paris. Yet it's a beefy Royal Canadian Mounted Policeman — in full battle regalia, sans cheval — who salutes me at the door. Where am I, anyway? Could it be that the bottle of burgundy I've consumed is playing parlor games with my mind? "No, not at all," says the smiling coatcheck lady. "Welcome to ze Crazy Horse, ze sexiest cabaret in all of Paree."

No one will ever mistake ze Crazy Horse for Amsterdam's Bananenbar. Red is the predominant color here, and not a whorehouse red, either. The walls and ceilings are lacquered a rich red, and the seats in the intimate Crazy Horse theater are covered in plush red velour. A little tacky, yes, but somehow tasteful — dare we even say refined? So, check any unsavory thoughts with your coat and go inside to see how civilized Parisians can be when they feel like it. As do most European adult-oriented revues, The Crazy Horse caters primarily to relatively upper-crust couples. The wild-eyed voyeurs, spittle dangling, are encouraged to get their jollies at the hard-core porn shows in Pigalle.

There are plenty of cabarets in Paris. There is the Moulin Rouge, immortalized by Toulouse Lautrec and famed for its high-kicking cancan dancers. And the equally colorful Paradis Latin and Lido revues, with their legions of knockout strutters. But The Crazy Horse, situated in the chic Eighth Arrondissement, has a cachet all its own. To scores of cash-rich tourists from around the globe, The Crazy Horse epitomizes all that is naughty and nice about Paris. We're talking major babes here — arguably the most gorgeous in the world. Founded in 1951 by artist and antiques-dealer Alain Bernardin, The Crazy Horse was conceived as a showcase for "l'art du nu" (the art of the nude — only the French could get away with a catchall term like that without making the cynics snicker); and the club has been upholding that mandate ever since.

Tonight's show is titled, appropriately, *Teasing*. The opening number is "God Save Our Bareskin," and, as with all the numbers in the show, the title is far more risqué than the actual content. Twelve ladies march out onto the stage wearing big, furry Beefeater chapeaus and little else. What's remarkable about them is not that they're virtually naked, but that they all appear to have been cast from the same mold. Their firm breasts and buttocks, even their faces, are almost identical. If cloning will be standard practice in the brave new world of tomorrow, then by all means let's start here. Yes, science can be our friend.

These lovely performers clearly possess a cheeky sense of humor. One can only assume they weren't born with the following monickers: Chica Boum, City Nebula, Fuzzy Logic, Izy Corridor, Jennifer De Lance, Lola Fragola, Loulou Looping, Pussy Duty-Free, Roxy Tornado, Sara Pimlico, Sleepy Nightmare, and Xenia Zigzag. Still, though their names conjure up the sort of antics you might expect from such American porno stars as Serenity and Slutwoman, rest assured that the kinkiest the Crazy Horse ladies get is doing stretching exercises on a hula hoop (as demonstrated by the remarkably flexible Ms. Roxy Tornado during another number). The emphasis is all on class here. When was the last time you went to a strip club and heard a patron comment, "Man, is this lighting ever awesome!" Yet such is the sort of repartee one overhears all the time at The Crazy Horse. There is not an iota of sleaze to be found.

Hard to believe that in a bygone era this stuff was considered sinful. Times change. Nowadays, you could escort your granny to The Crazy Horse and she wouldn't even flinch. She's seen and heard far more on the tube. But this doesn't mean that the cabaret's mannered elegance isn't suggestive. According to aficionados, the beauty of The Crazy Horse is that it does leave so much to the dark recesses of the imagination, which is precisely the way the French seem to like it in ze boudoir. One of the revue's showstoppers is an understated piece in which a performer is seen — stripping off her fishnet stockings with the help of one of her shoes. It's the sort of routine that could be used to warm up the crowd for a little crooning from Frank Sinatra and his Rat Pack. The same could be said of the performance of a shadowed woman who provocatively peels off her clothing while stretched out in a recliner chair.

A retired and seemingly unfulfilled American gentleman sitting next to me gets his hopes up when he hears that the next act is to be interpreted by Vik and Fabrini. He's convinced, he tells me, that Vik and Fabrini are a couple, possibly two women, who will shake things up by making love onstage. Imagine, then, this gentleman's surprise and disappointment when he discovers that Vik and Fabrini are a Brazilian prop comic and a sidekick mime. They are both guys, to boot, and their shenanigans are completely harmless. Nor is The Crazy Horse's Buka some electrifying belly dancer who lets it all hang out. Rather, Buka is a male magician who speaks an Arab dialect and does card tricks. Of course, Buka is, without question, the kinkiest act of the night, because although he's fully clothed, he appears to be pulling playing cards out of his butt, crotch, and ears. Life can be cruel. If Buka were a babe, he could bring his act to the Bananenbar and strike it rich; instead, he must endure yawning tourists who come to The Crazy Horse expecting to witness so much more than the three of spades emerging from a magician's ear.

Understand that after the no-holds-barred antics of Amsterdam's sex artistes, almost anything pales by comparison. Even the pig-dogs who populate Paris's famous Pigalle district look a little pallid. I'm confused. So off I go to visit my old pal Fabien. He'll set me straight. Fabien only appears to be a waiter at the Bofinger brasserie adjacent to Paris's grand Place de la Bastille. In fact, the friendly Fabien is, like most of his fellow country-men, an unpaid philosopher. Sometimes it's hard to understand how Fabien can carry his tray, for he is already laden with vital factoids and all manner of statistics on the human condition.

"Do you prefer to get or to give sexual pleasure?" Fabien asks, while pouring the Pouilly Fumé. But before I can open my yap and utter something profound, he indicates that I am not actually meant to answer this question. He's building up to a pronouncement about the French in general. He goes on to explain that in a recent French poll, sixty percent of women said they preferred to get sexual pleasure, while only forty per-cent of men stated the same preference. Fabien suggests that this amounts to a stunning reversal of what a similar survey might have deduced decades earlier. I ask him what his point is, and he stammers, "Don't you see? The men of France are be-coming women." By that, Fabien doesn't mean transgendered; he means sensitive. "Yes, and the women are becoming virile," he adds. By that, Fabien doesn't mean they're scratching their crotches in public; he simply means that they are expressing their sexual needs. So what does it all amount to? Says Fabien, with pride, "Frenchmen are the best lovers in the world, as sur-vey after survey proves. We were created to care for, and serve, our women. There is no more noble calling."

Well and good, but, garçon, there is a fly in my brains — er, my plate of ris de veau. When the fly has been extricated, Fabien and I discourse on the uniqueness of Paris when it comes to matters of the heart. Certainly, smut flourishes in Paris.

Check out St. Denis, Bois de Boulogne, and, of course, Pigalle, and you'll uncover a full range of sexual expression. You'll also find humor. I'm sorry, but eighty-year-old hookers practicing their profession in the comfort of their Peugots parked in the Bois constitutes comedy. And check out the upper echelons of government, where you'll find all kinds of sex scandal. But Paris oozes so much romance that it tends to offset the sleaze and the scandal. Far from being revolted, the French perceived an element of romance in the recent disclosure that deceased head of state François Mitterand would regularly entertain three different women in an evening, none of whom were his wife or numero-uno mistress.

In the words of a few fellow Dofinger diners — some wise, young Belgian designers in the employ of fashion darling Ann Demeulemeester — in this part of the world, sex is all about dressing things up, not stripping them down. It's about leaving it to the imagination. More can be more, say designers Ludi and Miriam over glasses of Veuve Cliquot. The human form is divine, but it can be even more divine when it is fashionably swathed in bold colors and textures. Some say the so-called French paradox has to do with the French being able to swill wine and feast on foie gras without falling victim to clogged arteries and heart attacks. Others, however, maintain that the French paradox is related to the idea that sex appeal comes from clothing. To gather further proof, the Demeule-meester design team suggests that I go to the Louvre and catch a prêt-à-porter fashion show. Waiter/philosopher Fabien agrees: "Anyone can take their clothes off. That's not difficult. And it's not always erotic to see what is under the clothing. Ahh, but it is a real art to put on clothes and it can definitely be erotic watching a fully clothed woman."

So it's off to the world of haute couture in my quest to gain more insight into humanity and sex. Many of the other people who have come to this auditorium in the Louvre are eager to see designer Karl Lagerfeld's autumn-winter collection for

Chanel. Still others are eager to spot celebrities. They aren't disappointed: Oscar nominee Julianne Moore, the unsinkable Tracey Ullman, and the captivating Carole Bouquet are among the luminaries who have squeezed themselves into the venue. It's clear that this is an event of earth-shattering proportions, because there are hundreds of photographers on hand. But, like everyone else, the photogs are getting restless. They are perched precariously atop their camera cases and are not amused that the spectacle commences a good forty-five minutes late. Some have had to stake their positions more than three hours earlier, all for the privilege of snapping some moppet in a shmata. Their photos aren't even likely to make it into a newspaper or magazine you or I will ever see.

No matter. This is like a big-ticket rock show. The designers and their models are superstars as huge as any pop icon. The atmosphere is electric as the show kicks off. A Madonna tune blares as models stream along the runway. In their puffy white parkas and heavy red lipstick, they strut and they pout. Their hair has been carefully mussed; cowlicks strategically conceal half their faces. This is not so much about fashion, it's about attitude. Unlike strippers, models never smile. They frown the frown of a person suffering from an excess of intestinal gas. They look like hookers going about their duties with the utmost reluctance. And yet they strike just the right note. Which is to say, they evoke desire. They make their turtlenecks and skirts and pants and parkas come off cool and funky and sexy in a kind of eighties retro way. Taking their cue from Madonna's "Vogue," they "pose" as the singer commands them.

In all, ninety models have participated in this stream-of-fashion-consciousness blur, leaving much of the audience breathless. Ullman numbers among those who've gone ga-ga over Karl Lagerfeld. "I just loved it," she gushes. "I kept nudging my husband and going, 'Christmas, Christmas, birthday, birthday.'" Backstage, the man himself manipulates his trademark fan, appearing to blow off the warmth and kudos that are flowing his way. Everyone tells Lagerfeld that he's a genius. He's heard it all many times before. He doles out sound bites: "My girls all have attitude and they have energy. But I'm always on the lookout for new girls." Someone tells him that his designs are just so modern. He seems perplexed. "I don't know what 'modern' means. I just know what feels right for the moment. My clothes are not about luxury. People can wear them like they wear jeans."

Since any type of inanity seems to fly here, this fashion expert sticks his neck out and asks Karl if he strives for that chic, sexy look. Karl rewards me with the same look he bestows on everyone else, like I've just blown in from some farflung locale where there are no fashion police. "I don't know," he says irritably, fanning himself a little harder. "I just design. This is clothing for the woman back in her hotel waiting for her lover to return." Ah, now I understand. I then ask, "What about your penchant for the music of Madonna, Karl?" That's easy. "I love a woman over forty who reinvents herself all the time without looking ridiculous." Obviously spoken by someone who hasn't seen a Madonna movie lately.

A scrum of reporters has now encircled and captured Karl Lagerfeld, so I drift away and approach André Leon Talley, *Vogue*'s larger-than-life fashion-editor-at-large. "Chanel is altissimo, darling," he coos. "It has everything for the new woman. It is Chanel's best collection yet. It is risky yet restrained. This is clothing for everyone from eighteen to eighty, and it's so appropriate that we are seeing it in Paris, the City of Light, the City of Creativity." "Well and altissimo, André, but would you say these duds are sexy, exuding allure?" Inquiring minds need to know why I've come to this fashion show to get the skinny on erotica. "Yes," André replies, "but not vulgar. Flirty sexy with a sense of sophistication. There is a noblesse d'esprit, a wit and a poetry to this line."

With all this gushing, with all the bon mots being bandied about, it's easy to lose sight of the fact that we're talking skirts here — not rocket science. Again, only in Paris can folks gurgle up any old non-sequitur and make it sound ever so sexy and occasionally even meaningful. If I, however, should return home and tell my buddies they're "altissimo" and praise their "noblesse d'esprit," I'll be banished for life.

Franco Rossi is a veteran of the fashion wars. For thirty-one years, he has been snapping away at fashion shows in Paris, Milan, and Tokyo. One of the best and most respected photogs in the biz, he represents two dozen newspapers and magazines around the world, including *Cosmopolitan*, *Vogue*, and the *Los Angeles Times*. And is he blown away by all the glitz? Not in the least. It's work. And it's stressful. Fashion photographers are forever on the go. They have to worry about lighting and positioning and getting a decent shot and covering their costs. As a consequence, they generally chug magnums of Maalox, not champagne. While Rossi has also taken pictures in some of the world's more volatile political climates, he insists that the fashion milieu is far more difficult and dangerous. Hell, you could lose an eye at a fashion show when all those photogs start jockeying for position.

"But surely," I innocently ask, "isn't it all worth it if you get to shoot some of the world's most beautiful and desirable women?" Rossi doesn't know whether to impale me with his tripod or simply walk away. Instead, he decides to bear with me. "Fifteen years ago, the work was fun, because the models were more professional. Now they take any fifteen-year-old kid. They aren't even trained. Some are so clumsy that they end up walking like cows and fall off the runway. At least hookers know how to walk and are more conscious of the image they project. Some of these models just don't have a clue." In the good old days, Rossi maintains, photographers had a great rapport with the models, but that's all changed. Blame it on the Naomi Campbell phenomenon, he says. "Designers pay her a fortune to model their clothes, and she poses with her eyes shut and her head turned. She just doesn't care." Rossi prefers a model like Pat Cleveland. "It didn't matter what she looked like. She simply brought life to whatever clothes she happened to be wearing. Today's models look like clothes hanging on the dry-cleaner's rack, rotating around with no feeling at all. And yet they think they are such stars. Just because you give a camera to some guy on the street doesn't mean he's a photographer. And just because you put some girl on a runway doesn't mean she's a model."

If you listen closely at a fashion show, you might hear the photographers emit sounds you'd expect to hear at the Grand Prix. That's their way of telling the models they're walking too fast to be photographed. "What designers forget is that people forget their designs half an hour after the show has ended," notes Rossi. "That's why they need our photos, to remind people." Rossi used to date models. Now he passes. He can deal with self-absorption and even airheadedness, but he can't deal with a lack of professionalism. Besides, models of the moment see themselves as movie stars and are mostly interested in bedding bona fide screen idols, rock legends — or one another.

Due to its mercenary aspect, some compare modeling to the world's oldest profession. Girls in both fields are in it mainly for the money. All the same, Rossi bristles at the suggestion that some modeling agencies are little more than escort services. He says, "There have always been girls with some agencies who've never made it as top models but who have resorted to other means to make money. It doesn't mean the fashion world is more corrupt than any other business. It just means that there are some greedy people here who will do what they can to get ahead, as is the case in many other lines of work." Or, as the Hungarian porn star Mercedes so succinctly put it in *Nerve* magazine, "I never thought I'd go into porn, but it's better than modeling. If you model, you have to have sex with the agent, the booker, and the photographer. In porn, I only have to have sex with one person." And I'm suddenly reminded of some words of wisdom I heard Bill Margold utter in Las Vegas: "In Hollywood, you have to screw to get the part. In X-rated films, you only have to screw after you get the part. But at least you know what you're getting yourself into."

Leaving the flighty world of fasion, we enter the combat zone. On Paris's Left Bank, a battle has long been waged against censorship. In the late fifties and early sixties, French publisher Claude Tchou stuck his neck out so that others could enjoy the freedom to print and sell literature which the forces-that-be had deemed unacceptable. Tchou challenged the law and became the country's first publisher, in this period, to stamp his company's imprint on erotic literature and sell it openly in the bookstores. For his efforts, he was actually sentenced to three months in prison, but the conviction was eventually overturned. Tchou is a most dignified and erudite man, and he doesn't think of himself as the pioneer who paved the way for porno in France. For him, it's all been about personal freedoms and his own love of literature. Tchou believes that people should at least have the right to choose whether they want to read *Sade* or *The Story of O*, among other books his company has published. "Under Charles de Gaulle's regime," states Tchou, "we were imposed with his nineteenth-century values and his bourgeois notions regarding censorship. It was not only books that were judged to be erotic that were banned, but also books that happened to have a few erotic passages. It was absurd. Someone had to take a stand."

Tchou could have done what others in this field did, which was to publish erotica under a pseudonym and deal only on the black market, but he felt that would be hypocritical. "What started to concern me even more was that authors began to censor themselves in their writing for fear of recrimination," he says. "When that happens, we're in a very sorry state."

Oddly, Tchou's interest in erotica was fueled by his friendship with author Henry Miller. The two talked about Tchou publishing Miller's collected works, but the author balked because he felt it was premature. "He insisted he should be dead before his complete works were published," Tchou notes. Another factor that motivated Tchou to publish erotica was aesthetics. It galled him that erotic literature was being published in a shoddy manner and was rife with grammatical errors. Be it Sade or Shakespeare, the meticulous Tchou can only abide finished products that are top-of-the-line, from paper quality to fonts to bibliographies. He published more than eighty volumes of erotica that had been "incarcerated in the hell" of France's Bibliothèque Nationale. Now, censorship of erotica is almost nonexistent in France. "I wasn't looking to make a footnote for myself in the history books," explains Tchou, who also credits French publisher Eric Losfeld with being a leader in the struggle against literary censorship. "I just felt the laws weren't in tune with the times. Really, boy meets girl and they make love — it is so normal. In the sixties, the sexual revolution was taking place in the West. And we were hardly Mormons or Quakers in France, but the laws made it seem that way."

You might expect that Tchou would be impressed with the proliferation of porno in the United States. You would be wrong. "America is still such a puritanical society," he says, echoing the sentiments of the Hef. "Sure, pornography is flourishing, but not erotica. And for me, that's a different thing altogether. I find much of the pornography vulgar and boring. If you've seen one, you've seen ten; and if you've seen ten, you've seen them all. More to the point, maybe there's no censorship in the U.S., but it is still a Republican society that executes people, and that is pornography when it comes down to it."

Tchou is out of the field of erotica now. He is publishing previously out-of-print books on everything from wine to psychology and marketing them through the Internet. But his views haven't mellowed over the years. "Censorship is a horrible thing. It's antidemocratic. It's fascist. Not just as it pertains to erotic literature, but to everything. The government has no business sticking its nose into the business of books and deciding what should be published. If someone decides to publish a manual about how to commit suicide or something on child pornography, you can assume this is an evil person, but it's up to the public whether or not they should buy it. And should someone actually kill themselves as a result of reading a self-help manual about suicide, then the publisher and author should be prosecuted for contributing to this. But that's not censorship. That's about committing a crime."

It should be noted that Tchou's greatest contribution to culture wasn't winning the battle against literary censorship in France, but rather in getting his fellow countrymen to read. A Parisian Oprah, if you will. He was instrumental in launching the Book of the Month Club in France, as well as the Rare Book Club, the History Book Club, the Book Club for Young Readers, and, of course, the Erotic Book Club. Meeting men like Tchou starts to make one feel better about the human condition.

Back at the Bofinger, the ever-helpful Fabien maintains that no treatise on sex would be complete without the wisdom of Picasso, who fought his share of battles against the moral authority and who was consumed with women and eroticism. In lieu of a meeting with the man himself (he passed away in 1973), Fabien suggests a quick jaunt over to the Musée Picasso at the Hôtel Salé in the Marais district. Although born in Spain, Picasso came to Paris as a young man at the turn of the twentieth century and, like many before him, he was seduced by the city. The museum created in his honor houses only a small percentage of Picasso's paintings, drawings, sculptures, and prints, but its collection clearly conveys the artist's vision and his obsession with women. *Nu Couché, Nu Assis, Nu Débout. Nu Couché Avec Personnages. Trois Nus.* You get the picture. Picasso, as art experts have pointed out, is not merely content to depict beautiful women; he explores them in all their unique nakedness. Of his scores of models, muses, lovers, and friends, seven women had such a profound effect on the artist's life that their names designate distinct periods of his work: Fernande, Eva, Olga, Marie-Thérèse, Dora, Françoise, and Jacqueline. According to Picasso authority Anette Robinson, every time a new woman came into his life, he changed his style. Picasso wanted each of his women to serve as mother, friend, muse, lover to keep his creative flame burning. In return, Picasso offered them unbridled passion and, eventually, a place in some of the world's finest museums and private collections.

A visitor to the Musée Picasso could spend hours in a reverie, gazing at the artist's tender *Portrait of Olga in an Armchair*. Picasso was clearly smitten with Olga Kokhlova, whom he met in Rome when she was there dancing with the Ballets Russes. She posed for him. They married in 1919, and Picasso's life was transformed — until the next woman came along. As entrancing as his portraits of Olga, Françoise, Dora Maar, and Jacqueline are, Picasso is just as capable as shocking — with, for example, the richly colored but grotesquely disjointed *Woman in an Armchair*. Picasso was as provocative as he was unpredictable. The poet Paul Eluard, a close friend of the artist, once commented: "Picasso loves intensely, but he kills what he loves."

My friend Fabien says Picasso was an enigma who understood the power of love in a way that few people ever have and, consequently, loved like few others ever have. Fabien also says he was a pretty fair artist, too.

It's so easy to be swept away by the romance, the art, the food, the fashion, and even some of the friendly waiters of Paris that one loses sight of the city's darker side. Porno in Paris? Sure, it exists. The French have taken up in-line skating with a vengeance. It is not pretty. It is not romantic. It is not remotely erotic. You might say it verges on the pornographic. Parisians may be dynamite in the sack and look dynamite outside of it, but they have to be the most spastic rollerbladers on the planet. The world's most beautiful women, their men, and their children, risk life and limb every weekend on a makeshift track at the Place de la Bastille. They crash into the customers and — horrors — the waiters at the outdoor cafés, because they haven't mastered the fine art of smoking a cigarette, conducting a cell-phone conversation, and in-line skating simultaneously. Fabien is naturally appalled, since he has endured more than his fair share of bruises inflicted by errant rollerbladers. But he has a ready explanation: "It's the Big Guy's way of evening things out in the world. Really, we can't have everything. It would be unjust that the world's greatest lovers would also be the best skaters." Fabien ain't fooling.

So, where's the filth? It's there. It's like that French flick *Une Liaison Pornographique*, starring Nathalie Baye and Sergi Lopez. It tells the story of a fantasy-starved couple who live in Paris and meet through a personal ad. The two pursue pornographic adventures together, but — get this — they end up falling in pure love instead. The film's title turns out to be a misnomer, just as the very concept of porno, for many Parisians, like that hardcore romantic Fabien, turns out to be something else entirely. My unpaid philosopher friend offers more counsel: "Go to the colonies," he tells me. "That's where all the action is today." When he says "colonies," Fabien is not referring to the United States. He is referring to the French-speaking colony of Quebec, a Canadian province that has preserved its Gallic charm and attitude and permissiveness, but that is actually still a part of the British Commonwealth. "The women are even more beautiful and more wild than here," Fabien enthuses. "And the men are far better rollerbladers." Well, that clinches it. Garçon, mon avion!

Chapter 6

TWO TONGUES ARE BETTER

MONTREAL

Into diapers and disco? Still continent? Well, do we have a party for you. It's Fetish Night at Montreal's cavernous Club Cream, setting of the city's shiniest masquerade ball. There is a proviso, though: apart from those sporting diapers, only folks in rubber, latex, and vinyl, preferably toting whips, cuffs, chains, and canes, are permitted to attend Fetish Night. A Montreal S&M tradition since 1993, Fetish Night takes place the first Saturday of every month. And, without fail, more than five hundred patrons chomp at the bit to play, dance, grind, tie, tease, please, and spank.

Just about everything goes at Fetish Night. Save actual sex. Johnny Sardelli, the mastermind behind these soirées, has a surprisingly strict value system for someone who makes his daily bread selling spiked dog collars, thigh-high boots, and whips. "I encourage people to look and touch, but intercourse is absolutely forbidden," says the shirtless, leather-pants-wearing Sardelli, while greeting customers at the door of Club Cream. "Oh, yes, and I insist people stay true to their marriage vows."

Sardelli does. His wife is featured in the brochures and advertising for Il Bolero, Sardelli's Montreal fetish emporium.

Bolero was Montreal's first fetish shop, and it is still considered the ne plus ultra by those in the latex know. Sardelli insists that his is not a sex shop but, rather, a high-end fetish fashion store. He caters to the carriage trade — judges, doctors, stockbrokers, physicists — and sells just about everything but bridles, although he can arrange for those, too. A year after opening Bolero, Sardelli realized he had an interesting dilemma on his hands. The people who were stocking up on all his party fetish gear had no place to show it off; and, as Sardelli can attest, those who favor fetish gear live to exhibit their wares. So Fetish Night was born. Sardelli started modestly on the first Monday of the month, then on the Thursday, and finally, because of the demand, made it the Saturday. Although he could probably pack the place weekly, he has opted to make the party a monthly affair in order to maximize its impact. He sees the evenings as something akin to therapy for the overimaginative. "Fetish Night is all about people fulfilling fantasies," he says. "It's a place where people respect one another and never judge." In short, an S&M paradise.

Word of Sardelli's soirées has spread far and wide. Rubber-souled tourists from New York, Toronto, and Europe make a point of being in Montreal on Fetish Night. Even my Parisian friend Fabien has heard incredible tales about this Fetish Night. Sardelli laps it all up. "Ten years ago, this would have been unthinkable," he says. There were taboos against this sort of thing. Now, no one raises an eyebrow. We have no problems with the police, because we obey the law — which is to say we don't allow intercourse in the club." Drugs, too, are verboten, but the booze flows and the music blares. "When we first started, people would come to either dominate or to submit," he notes. "But now it's much more relaxed." Sardelli's family is fully supportive of his endeavors. "It's work. It's legal. It's money," he remarks. His wife used to work as a paralegal for the Canadian government's Department of Immigration, but she left her job to lend a hand at Bolero. Sardelli's brother also toils for the family firm.

Sardelli insists that Montreal is now a center for cutting-edge sexuality. "The only problem with this city is that there aren't enough dominatrixes" (back of the class and a spanking for those who thought he was going to say low-income housing). But no time for philosophizing now. It's about eleven o'clock at night. Club Cream's smoke machine is cranked. So is the music. And so are the patrons. I'm sitting at the bar next to a congenial couple. One half of the unit is attired in a smart pair of rubber pants; her significant other wears a leather skirt. The dude in the skirt is a bespectacled, fiftysomething dentist, and his rubber-clad wife is a research technician at a hospital lab. Take away their rubber and leather, and they could pass for the suburban couple next door. "We come here because we can fantasize without feeling guilty," he says. She simply nods and pinches his butt.

Next to me on the other side are a pair of lawyers in latex — matching ensembles, in fact. Again, remove the outerwear and you've got one very straight-looking couple. Behind the bar is Marie-Belle, who insists, not surprisingly, that she feels quite comfortable at Fetish Night. Says the enchanting bartender, "I love eccentrics and, better still, I love eccentrics who tip well." On the subject of great-tipping eccentrics, a short, stoutish, white-haired fellow, evidently a prominent university professor, shows off his garb to Marie-Belle. He's come as a Boy Scout, except that the shirt and shorts of his uniform are rubber. His friend, another elderly fellow, looks marvelous in a French-maid's getup — dress, apron, and duster.

At first, the scene is somewhat akin to a high school sock hop. People check out people from the sidelines and wait for someone to break the ice, to dance, and to prance. "It's kind of cute the way these people are so shy at first," muses Marie-Belle. "They want to cruise, but they don't want to be the first on the floor." At the first Fetish Night Marie-Belle worked as a bartender, she wondered why it was that she felt so safe in an environment that encourages people to give full rein to their dark sides. She's still wondering. "I feel safer here than I do at the supermarket," she says. "Funny, eh? But these are people who live to fantasize. No one gets hurt here." I'm starting to think this will be about as kinky as a church picnic, but Marie-Belle reassures me: "Just wait until the alcohol kicks in. Then they really loosen up."

And, sure 'nuf, Marie-Belle is right. Two minutes later, a preppie student type in leather underwear and tanktop takes to the stage and starts gyrating. He is joined by a guy in yellow rubber overalls with a gas mask over his mouth. They dance. They get the crowd going. The place starts to jump. And then the guy in the yellow overalls decides he wants a cigarette, but for a moment he forgets that he's wearing a gas mask. This produces jocularity in certain quarters. The guy in the gas mask recovers, though, and spanks his buddy with a pair of construction gloves. "Ow!" blurts his buddy. "What did you do that for?" Get with the program, dude.

Another couple saunters onto the floor. They are among the most wholesome-looking people I've ever seen. He's blonde. So is she. And, I'm sorry, but even in their matching leather lederhosen they look more like poster people for Hitler Youth than agents of Sodom. The music has gone beyond loud. It shakes my intestines. The dentist is dancing in a frenzy. He's sweating bullets, and consequently asks his bride to remove his studded dog collar. "I can't breathe," he screams. Neither can the guy in the gasmask, so he slips the thing off and lets it dangle from his neck. A ponytailed gentleman in a cage, wearing nothing but an apron, starts to do chin-ups to the beat of the music. "You really have to enter a trancelike state to get into this," Marie-Belle informs me. A young man who could pass for a preacher, were it not for the leather pants with handcuffs protruding from the pocket, approaches a young woman in a mask and Victorian-style corset, bows, and asks for the honor of a dance.

On the dance floor a strobelight distorts images, but only to a point. A skinny fellow in a tight-fitting leather corset, who looks like a wigged-out British glam-rock star from the seventies, is studiously observing a couple of women who are suggestively bopping to the technobeat. "There's little in the way of small talk here, so everything is left to the imagination," Marie-Belle pipes up. That's because the decibel level is such that not even an air-raid siren could penetrate it. Besides, Fetish Night was conceived as an outlet for exhibitionism, not a forum for deep thoughts. And, to be honest, who really wants to eavesdrop on an All-American linebacker-type in diapers as he whispers sweet nothings to a fellow dressed up as Marie Antoinette?

Now, one would imagine that it would be awfully difficult to stand out in a joint where rubber shorts are de rigueur and no one thinks anything of a poseur in Pampers, or a chubby, middle-aged man in a leather bra who is a dead ringer for *Seinfeld*'s George Costanza. After all, everyone is here to make a statement. But none more so than a statuesque blonde chick in leather — she does manage to make an impression. She must be about nine-foot-six in her elevator sandals. She towers over everyone, and some of us are a little concerned that she'll stomp on our toes with that killer footwear. She decides to dance at the bar, but mercifully not on top of it, and all of a sudden she's surrounded by The Village People, or a reasonable facsimile. One of The Village People attempts to initiate a conversation with Stretch (as I've dubbed the Amazon). "So what's doing?" he screams into the din. "Yeowwww!" retorts Stretch. "Nice getup," he retorts. "Yeowwww!" Stretch counters. "Wanna drink?" he asks. "Yeowwww!" Stretch replies. There's something a little fishy about Stretch, observes Andrea, looking demure in a latex dress. The shirtless Tarzan, with whom Andrea is shimmying, agrees. "I've got it," Andrea announces. "She's a he." Says Tarzan: "That's adorable." To which Stretch graciously answers, "Yeowwww!" Tarzan pulls out a whip and, with a little flick to Andrea's derriere, makes sign language to signify he'd like to dance with her again. Andrea, who's in the midst of chugging a brew, flashes Tarzan the sort of look that suggests she doesn't appreciate being whipped while drinking.

Rachel wanders up to the bar and apologizes for the way she's dressed to anyone who will listen. She is merely wearing dark clothing — a no-no. But Rachel has an excuse. She's just come from work; she does payment processing for some new-wave dot-com company. "The last Fetish Night, I came in a latex pantsuit and a blonde wig," she says. "It was a blast. Now I've come as me, someone who just wants to dance and forget about a horrendous relationship I just finished." Upon reflection, Rachel says she is drawn to these evenings, "because you can be whoever you want to be — even yourself." How's that for a concept? "Everybody is unique unto themselves here. Nobody is better or worse." And the conversations you overhear at Fetish Night can be priceless. To wit, the one between the masked Chandra and a fellow in a leather loincloth:

Him: "Who are you? I know you from somewhere."
Her: "No, you don't know me."
Him: "Yes, I do. Who are you?"
Her: "Who do you want me to be?"
Him: "Someone who will dominate me, but with that kind of attitude, I don't think you're the one."

Bummer. Chandra is starting to think she's come to some kind of disco-support-group soirée. "It doesn't feel very S&M," she complains. "Sure, people act out their fantasies on the dance floor, but it all feels so sanitized, almost like a family dinner. It's more about fashion than fetishes." Alas, Chandra may have spoken too soon. When she takes to the floor for a little free-shaking, she is immediately sandwiched by two guys dressed in leather from head to toe. They engage in some dirty dancing. Even more dirty than meets the eye, as it turns out.

Chandra emerges from this writhing mass sounding even more disappointed. "One of the guys imploded in his leather pants after rubbing on my knee," she sighs. "Oh my, I think we have a dry-clean situation here." She points to some unsightly spots on her latex dress. "Bad enough that I borrowed this dress from a friend, but then the guy acts like nothing has happened and innocently says, 'Hi, my name is David.' And all I can do is to say, 'Hi, my name is Chandra.'" Okay, *Love Story*, this ain't. But it's a start.

Meanwhile, for no apparent reason, I myself am dancing, solo, to a techno tune that appears to go like this: "Free your mind and your ass will follow." And I'm thinking it would be best if I exited now. I've very nearly been impaled on someone's six-inch spiked neck collar. Furthermore, Stretch is trashed and out of control on the dance floor, just about crushing the lawyer couple in latex — which, granted, might well be construed as a public service. On my way out the door, Rachel informs me that no self-respecting sex odyssey would be complete without a probe of Montreal's burgeoning porno-film biz. That's an order, she adds. So I'd best take heed.

First, a little background info on the adult film industry: few of the principals use their real names in the credits. This factoid comes courtesy of Lindsay Scott, communications director for Montreal-based Slinky Productions, the hot new kid on the adult entertainment block. To illustrate his point, Slinky's PR man explains that his name is really Scott Lindsay, which clearly doesn't have the same cachet as his pseudonym. In any event, Scott's revelation has spared me hundreds of hours of research. I had already scoured the film guides in vain, searching for the goods on Slinky's roster of stars — Tangerine Dream, Dolphin, Lexei Bacci, and resident stud Sonny Chase. One thing, however, is certain: Slinky is about to change the face of adult entertainment in Canada. (More background: in this age of euphemisms, Lindsay Scott, né Scott Lindsay, says the term *porno* is passé; producers now prefer the less-threatening term *adult* to describe this film genre.)

Slinky has just launched *Office Fantasies One: Behind the CEO*

Door, the first in a series of six bilingual (English and French) and bisexual adult films. In the debut tale, Bacci is cast as the lonely but lustful head of a marketing firm. But Bacci is not lonely for long. Not after encountering maintenance man Chase and job applicant Tangerine Dream. Then Dolphin dives into the fray, and it's a free-for-all. Okay, so the plot isn't up there with *The English Patient*'s, but the production values certainly surpass the Canadian film industry standard. All of this by way of saying that the flick wasn't shot in some dingy basement with an antique Super 8. In fact, as Scott proudly tells me, each film in the series has a budget of about fifty thousand dollars, which is three times the size of the average adult film budget. Scott also indicates that the films are shot with state-of-the-art digital Betacams and that the cameras are mounted on, er, dollies in an attempt to achieve realism and better depth of field. The names of the principals may have been changed, but all hail from Montreal and environs, and all are committed to infusing an element of style into this oft-maligned movie genre.

Slinky has already secured a distribution arrangement for the series across Canada; American and European release deals are imminent. Remarks Scott, "The problem with porno before was that the wrong people were making it. It's time for a little taste." Taste, of course, is a relative thing, and prospective viewers should beware that *Behind the* CEO *Door* isn't exactly Bergman's *Persona*. Regardless, producer Trevor Wright admits that after renting "too many" adult flicks, he came to the realization that "we could make better films ourselves." So he hooked up with a buddy, director Mario Antonacci, who uses his real name and who has also acquired real experience on the conventional movie scene. Antonacci maintains that "The stuff that has been produced in this country over the last twenty years is so cheesy. It's not believable."

Wright and Antonacci undertook market research to identify the audience for the adult fare they wanted to produce. They quickly deduced that the big consumers of porno flicks these days are your average couples, not the prototypical trench-coat set. Furthermore, these people want class, credibility, and polish. Wright and Antonacci haven't had trouble finding sponsors who share their dream. Unlike traditional movie backers — beer, cola, and car manufacturers — their sponsors include adult-accessories supplier Il Bolero and the exotic dance clubs Wanda's, Solid Gold, and Downtown. This is appropriate, since many of the stars of the series cut their showbiz teeth, and then some, on Montreal's vaunted strip-club circuit.

Circuit veteran Tangerine Dream makes her movie debut in *Behind the CEO Door*, and she'll also star in the second installment of the series. "It's always been a fantasy of mine to have sex in front of a camera," she explains. "I'm not ashamed of doing what's natural. I'm proud of my body. But you can't be shy in this line of work." Lexei Bacci, the only cast member with previous adult film experience, doesn't mince words either: "I'm an exhibitionist, and I'm comfortable with my sexuality." No question. All the same, Scott would like to reassure people that everything is aboveboard at the Slinky production offices. That is, life doesn't imitate art in the company boardroom. "It's all business," he says. "Except on those occasions when Lexei shows up and tries to shake things up, like only she can."

The setting is now a nifty seventy-foot yacht equipped with all the options. We're cruising the St. Lawrence River. The Slinky gang has gathered today for the shooting of the second *Office Fantasy* flick. Five men and five women performers are aboard, as are scores of media reps, who are happy to soak up a bit of sex from the sidelines. The hired studs, most of them neophytes, look somewhat apprehensive. It's hard enough to perform before a gaggle of onlookers, especially leering members of the media, but making matters worse is the fact that it's not exactly balmy out here on the deck. In the immortal words of Jerry Seinfeld's buddy George, "Shrinkage can be problematic." One of the actor-studs, Tino, while grateful for the opportunity to fulfill a fantasy, fears that he won't be able to perform on camera.

Lexei Bacci, naturally, has no such worries. She confesses that she never comes on camera — she only pretends to. "It's an act," she says with a broad smile. "I am an actress." Indeed, she is. When the camera is set up, the buxom Bacci rises to the occasion and fondles another female performer. Sadly, Tino isn't faring so well. Just as he had feared, he is not up to the task. Fortunately, Bruno, another rookie stud, is. He eagerly joins the melee.

Now it's director Mario Antonacci's turn to get antsy. He fears that Bacci is getting Bruno a tad *too* excited. "I need him for later," Antonacci pleads. And as if this scene isn't already surreal enough, a police schooner approaches the yacht. Most of us onboard are thinking bust, and we're not far wrong. But the cops seem content to gaze at Bacci's bust for a moment before their vessel moves off into the sunset.

The big moment has come. The producer barks instructions to his compliant cast: "Five minutes to showtime. Teeth brushed. Genitals washed. Guys, don't forget your condoms and K-Y. And don't forget to switch condoms every time you switch girls. And, oh yeah, if the camera isn't on you, go easy. It's a long day and I need to make it through." If you catch his drift. The boat begins to rock. A ten-person orgy can do this. Bacci is in her element. Bruno is pumped. Tino, too, is giving it the old college try. And then, wouldn't you know it, the rain starts falling and so do a few male appendages. The actors bolt for cover inside the cabin. "Very glamorous business, isn't it?" Bacci coos. "But that's showbiz." Fun's over for the media today.

Lexei Bacci, as advertised, can and does shake things up. A self-admitted accident waiting to happen, she inadvertently knocks over her cup of Spanish coffee and sprays everyone and everything within twenty feet. "I'm such a jinx. I feel terrible," she says, mopping up the spillage. Bacci is genuinely concerned. "Everything I touch, sometimes, spills." Well, yeah.

This is a rare day off for Bacci. We're sitting in the St. Viateur Bagel Café, home of the finest bagels in this solar system,

according to Montrealers. In fact, Montrealers will delight in
telling you that next to their women, their bagels are the most
scrumptious around. Bacci, true to her cultural roots, has
passed on the bagels and is munching a bunch of biscotti,
about the only items in the place that haven't been sprayed by
the Spanish coffee. Today, Bacci has reason to celebrate. She
has just launched her own Web site. She's just finished writing,
directing, producing, and starring in an adult film trilogy. And
she's just left the Slinky fold to establish the Bacci Mateo Empire. Bacci, who wears her platinum blonde hair cropped short
and is about to turn thirty, thinks in empire-like terms. It's re-
freshing. In bygone times, she would have been hanging with
the Caesars and cavorting with Caligula himself. Indeed, the
Roman Empire might still be standing if Bacci had been given
the run of the place.

Oddly, Bacci's trilogy is an ode to history — of sorts. The
first pic in the pack, *The Rise of Louis XVI*, is a manicured peek at
pomp in the boudoir of Marie Antoinette, who is played by
Bacci in a fetching powdered wig and related period attire. It's
the touching, if not entirely historically accurate, tale of the
king's attempts to make his way into Marie back in 1784, before
Ron Jeremy made his mark. Evidently, Marie is somewhat coy
— when it comes to Louis, anyway. Otherwise, she has an insatiable appetite. Knowing what he's up against, Louis disguises
himself as a masked peasant thief and bursts into Marie's boudoir, where he has his way with her, where she has her way
with him, and so on, and so on. Louis and Marie leave little to
the imagination in their desire to please one another.

"The element of sex, as such, is not that interesting," says
the articulate and always-candid Bacci. She is speaking more as
a director than as a performer, here. "It's been done to death.
It's the elements surrounding the element of sex that really
turn me on and that make for an interesting movie. Don't get
me wrong. After all, few love sex more than I do, but you have
to go beyond to interest viewers." Evidently sharing this view
are Bacci's masked costar, Ziggy Frost, and cinematographer

Satan Sands (Bacci doesn't even attempt to patronize me by revealing that these aren't their real names).

In the other two films of her series, Bacci pays equally close attention to period detail. *Climaxing Cleopatras*, starring Bacci in a dark wig and ancient Egyptian garb, features two Cleopatras climaxing often with one another. The flick is also a tribute to the strength and durability of the common cucumber. If they gave out porno Oscars to veggies, Bacci's cuke would be a shoo-in. There are no prominent parts for vegetables, however, in *Blondes Prefer Gentlemen*, the trilogy's final flick, in which Martha Washington — Bacci in stars-and-stripes regalia — shows her appreciation for men with manners. Clearly, Bacci loves sex, but at the end of each of her films a message is delivered: "Have sex. Have fun. Use condoms." She also makes it clear that all of the players in her films have been tested and are HIV-free.

Bacci has been around the adult video block in Canada and the U.S. She's been featured in at least fifty skin flicks, and likely far more, since many of the scenes she's filmed have become stock footage that is used in other oeuvres. It's safe to say that Bacci is one of the more experienced adult stars north of the Canada-U.S. border, and she's intent on maintaining an aura of professionalism in her work. The actors and technicians she employs are all experienced as well, but almost exclusively in mainstream movies, which helps to explain their need for aliases. For that matter, Bacci herself has appeared in some legit films, such as the Oscar-nominated saga *The Red Violin*. And she just may be one of the few porno stars anywhere who displays a penchant for performing the works of Molière. She's actually done it — fully dressed — on Montreal's legit theater stages. "That's why I am able to fake it so well in some of my sex scenes," she winks. "That's what classical theater training can do for you. It allows you to focus on the needs of other actors."

Onscreen, Bacci has engaged in every imaginable variety of sex with partners of both genders, but offscreen, she is one hundred percent hetero. "Before I got into the business, I used to fantasize about having sex and falling in love with women. But after having experienced this so often, I no longer fantasize and would be quite content in a monogamous relationship with a man." After spending time in Boston and Toronto, Bacci returned to her native Montreal in 1995, ostensibly to get married. But tensions arose between her and her longtime squeeze, an administrator in the construction trade, and they called off their nuptials. This prompted Bacci to take a total plunge into the porno biz: acting, writing, directing, and producing. "It's not always an easy balance," she explains. "While I really do get into the sex most of the time while I'm performing, the director part of me has to worry about the sets, lighting, focus, and the actors. I'm a perfectionist, and I'm the first to admit that directing is much more demanding than performing."

Bacci put about one hundred thousand dollars of her own money into her trilogy. She expects to recoup it through video sales and hits on her Web site. She sees that site as the glue that holds her porno cottage industry together. Not only does the site offer snippets of Bacci's greatest moves in the bedroom and the office, but it also has some decidedly nonkinky content. Click here to see Bacci pontificate on the latest — nonporno — films, T.V. shows, and CDs. She talks fashion — in fact, she retails her own line of clothing through the site's Bacci Boutique. She dispenses no-nonsense medical information about sexually transmitted diseases. She also has a chat room, where she allows Web surfers to unload their angst on her. Call her Dr. Lexei. Oh yeah, the site also features Bacci's original *Unhappy Hooker* cartoon series. The plight of hookers arouses feelings of empathy in Bacci. "Although I've never hooked, I find it funny that it's legal to have sex in front of a camera and get paid for it, but not when there is no camera around," she says. "I find it extremely hypocritical. Really, the moment you use your body to make money by having sex you're prostituting yourself. I'm under no illusions."

Not finished yet. With a couple of partners, Bacci also runs a bar in Montreal called La Petite Boîte. It's not what you're thinking. Says Bacci, "The place is so straight. You'd die. It's just regular working-class people, that's all." There is a method to the Bacci empire, and sex is only part of it. "So many people have underestimated me all my life," reflects Bacci. "They were all so certain that I'd flop no matter what I did. Maybe I will. But it won't be for a lack of trying. I've saved everything I've made and put it all back into the company." She didn't have to. She was making a good living before all this. She had no debts. "Sure, my life might have seemed perfect to some. But I was bored out of my mind. I thought I really wanted to settle down and lead a quiet life until I broke up with my fiancé. But sex has always been a large part of who I am. The problem was that few knew, certainly not my family and many of my friends. It was just becoming too heavy, forever hiding. But I couldn't live that way. Now people know. I feel better, but they were shocked. They had no clue. Most have come to accept me unconditionally for who I am. My father loves me, but he pretends that part of my life just doesn't exist. He still thinks of me as his innocent four-year-old daughter. He could not comprehend how his intelligent little girl, who loved theater and was always trying to better herself, could end up in this line of work. Telling him about my work was the hardest thing I've ever had to do in my life." Bacci's parents split up years ago. Bacci is estranged from her mother, but she maintains contact with her father and her only brother, with whom she has always been close. "My brother accepts my work, but he'd really like it if I could settle down and have a family. On the surface, that seems ideal, but I don't think I'm ready for that yet."

Bacci's father is a wedding photographer and her mother, says Bacci, hinting at the nature of their estrangement, "mostly spends money" and indulges herself. Though Bacci went to an exclusive private French school, dysfunctionality flourished on the homefront when she was growing up. Her parents were strict with her. Her teachers were also strict, and they tried to impose religion on her. She rebelled at an early age. "I think I had an inclination that I was going to be quite involved in sex way back in first grade," she says. "Even then, I was a bit of a sex maniac, fantasizing about little boys. I loved boys. But I kept up this charade of being virtuous at home until I was sixteen and finally left. Then I became very promiscuous. It was just pure sex I was after — not love. And it had nothing to do with drugs or alcohol. To this day, I don't drink, I don't smoke, and I don't do drugs. I'm actually quite straight in most respects. I want to see what's going on around me. My only addiction was, and is, sex." Bacci has never sought treatment. "Why ruin a good thing?" she quips. "Anyway, I was, and still am, in control. I don't hurt people. Sex has actually been the most honest part of my life. I don't hide behind barriers. On occasion, I'm unsure of myself intellectually, but I've always been sure of myself sexually. And I still want to explore. There's a ridiculous assumption made that women can't be intelligent and work in sex. What a joke. I'm here to prove I can be an exhibitionist as well as a damn smart businesswoman."

Besides, the sex is more than sex. "People stop clicking the channel when they see or hear sex," Bacci points out. "It's my opportunity to get a message across to women — that sexiness is not a look, it's an attitude. A woman can weigh one hundred or one hundred and eighty pounds — it doesn't matter. What matters is that women love themselves, that they not feel ashamed of their bodies, and that they explore all the pleasure sex has to offer. Hopefully, I can sell my brain as well as my butt in my films."

Suddenly, Bacci is Dr. Ruth. But that's enough philosophy for the time being. Wanna make Bacci howl with laughter? Ask her about the porno world's so-called marathon men. She rolls her eyes. "Ah, the magic of editing. What you see in the final cut and what actually transpired on the set are two different things." So let's cut to the chase. "Well, let's just say that it's very rare to find the stud who can get hard, stay hard, and come on command. Those who can master that are special indeed. To be fair to the other guys, though, the atmosphere around a shoot is not terribly sexy. It's more industrial. You've got publicists, media people, and crew running around. It doesn't matter how much the guy loves sex, he has to be so above what's going on around him to perform. The funny thing is that the women get paid more than the men in this business. It's not fair. A woman can slap on some K-Y jelly and she's ready to go. But a guy just can't fake it."

Bacci confesses that she's had to employ stunt studs to double for her leads on many occasions. In fact, one scene in her trilogy took three days to shoot and involved a variety of contributors. "Look — time is money," Bacci the producer states. "You can't wait for a guy forever to get excited. But at least I made sure there was continuity over those three days." Bacci praises her *Louis XVI* costar, Ziggy Frost. He had absolutely no experience in the field, she says, yet he performed like a total pro. As for Zig's mask, it was that or get fired from his day job. Evidently, Mr. Frost is an exec for some big-shot firm; it's unlikely that his bosses would be pleased if he became famous for his onscreen dive into Marie Antoinette's privates. Like Ziggy, many of those involved in Bacci's project are visitors to the porno world; and they're delighted to be there. "It's funny. The cinematographer, the editor, and all the other crew come from serious movie backgrounds, but they just love working this side of the business. There's a freedom and, of course, an intimacy."

The one thing that really gets Bacci steamed is the mere mention of child porno. In fact, most of the other porno-biz players I've encountered have a similar reaction. "As long as the actors are consenting and over eighteen," says Bacci, "it's okay. But I will not tolerate anyone who exploits children who have no clue what they're doing. That's a crime. And anyone who is involved deserves prison. No excuses." She also draws the line at animals. "I've been with a lot of men who were beasts. But I've never done it with any animal."

Bacci goes on to reveal that the best and wildest sex she's ever had with a man has been off the film set. "There's nothing more magical than real romance to bring out the best in sex."

None of this is to suggest that sex consumes Bacci entirely. She has other interests: photography, cooking, hiking, travel. And, of course, Molière. Her favorite Molière play is *Les Femmes Savantes*. "I would play the mother. I was always choosing the dominant roles. That's the control freak in me. But it's the live-audience aspect that made me love the theater so much. In front of a camera, it's boring, and it can be so easily faked. But everything is on the line onstage. There's so much more passion. If I had the time, I'd go back to the stage — even if the role called for lots of clothing that stayed on. I can be very flexible." Flexible enough to play Blanche Dubois in *A Streetcar Named Desire*. "She was sexually repressed, and I can relate to that. Even people like me in this business are repressed, because there are still so many more fantasies out there." Okay, I'll bite. What fantasies? "Don't laugh," she says, ever so innocently. "But sometimes when I'm alone at night, I wish I had someone lying next to me for some spontaneous romance. Ahh, deep down, I guess I'm an old-fashioned girl at heart."

Lexei Bacci doesn't bask in cheap sentiment for long. She has another film trilogy to play. This time, she's thinking gay male. "I just hope the set survives intact. Gee, even I broke the sofa twice in *The Rise of Louis XVI*. Can't imagine what a bunch of wild guys would do." Obviously, Bacci's writing herself out of such a series, and that's just fine with her. She'll retire from performing one of these days, and then she wants to focus more on the direction, writing, and production. "I've had a great run. I feel quite blessed to have lived my life the way I have and without shame. No regrets at all. When I was young, I dreamed of becoming a lawyer. I was naive. But it all worked out in the end. I wound up screwing people anyway." She winks. Takes a last nibble of her biscotti. And exits stage left.

So, what's whipped cream got to do with it? Not a whole bunch. There's not much in the way of whips, chains, or latex bodysuits, either, at the Salon de l'Amour et Séduction, which takes place annually at the Palais des Congrès, Montreal's not-especially-kinky convention center. Wanna new perspective on the brave new world? Then, by all means, get your glasses steam-cleaned at one of the salon's stalls.

Montreal is some kind of quirky town, and it's obsessed with sex. This particular luvvv salon, however, isn't really geared for the trench-coat brigade. It aims to demystify and "desmarm" sex, according to one insider. I wouldn't want to suggest that this affair is overly sanitized — after all, a bevy of Québécois porno queens is on hand for a signing-and-gawking session with their fans. But the innocent onlooker could easily come away with the impression that this is all about as titillating as a seminar on tax planning.

It's a far cry from Amsterdam's Bananenbar. You could bring your granny here. In fact, I've just met someone else's granny and grandpa. Mariette and Roger are typical salon visitors. Roger is a butcher, and Mariette is a "household technician." They're eyeballing a harness strong enough to bolster Montreal's infamous Olympic Stadium. "In the old days, sex was so hush-hush and was seen as a sin," remarks Mariette. "Now, everything is out in the open, as it should be." Interjects Roger, fifty-nine, "We've been married thirty-three years, and we're still curious. Even an old guy like me can learn." Roger and Mariette, who have three children and a couple of grandchildren, 'fess up to a fascination with porno videos. "As long as the stories are good, that is," adds Mariette.

Among those browsing through the salon are students, seniors, housewives, and sundry suburbanites — and, like the good burghers of Amsterdam, not one wears a lascivious grin. They've come to get the skinny on lotions, lingerie, and naughty things that go bang in the night. Thanks to the New Age musical stylings of Pan-flutist Bobaru — a student of the legendary Zamfir — the mood is so mellow that visitors could feel like curling up in a fetal position and catching forty winks rather than performing sexual calisthenics. Sure, a number of exhibitors are pushing some quirky products. Like penis pasta. "I'll have mine al dente," quips a matron.

Certainly, some could get their jollies examining French ticklers that glow in the dark or videos like *The Butt Sisters Do Daytona*, but even business in the small X-rated part of the salon is being conducted with dignity. Hell, the employees of Boutique Sexe Cité are traipsing about in tuxes. Pascal Harvey, the straightlaced manager of the boutique, tells me that China-brush sales are brisk. "To avoid premature ejaculation," explains the man in the tuxedo matter-of-factly. Boutique owner Alain St. Jacques begs to differ. "No, I think the lotions and lingerie are the big sellers," he says, before concluding, "Some people think just sick people go to sex shops. But in the ten years I've had my business, I've never met more regular people."

I move along, and soon I find myself passing a biorhythm booth — presumably for those delicate moments when the brain says, "Yes! Yes!" but the body says, "No way." Then it's over to Fantasia, where the friendly Maggie offers free slurps of a potion called Oil of Love. "No thanks," I say. "You can also rub it on certain body parts," she says. "Not now, thanks." According to the equally congenial Madelaine, Fantasia is a takeout service for folks who are too embarrassed to show their faces in a sex shop. The ladies of Fantasia — all married with kids — organize something akin to Tupperware (shtupperware?) parties with a Kama Sutra slant in their customers' homes. "What makes it work is that we're so normal," Maggie tells me. "Sometimes, even our husbands come along for the show," chimes in Madelaine, while demonstrating a minivibrator that hops. "Don't ever do this on a table," she warns. Fret not.

Next, it's over to the face-lift acupuncture stall. Then I check out the eyeglass-cleaning display. Whoa! Eyeglass cleaning? Salon of seduction? This does not compute. "If you want to see your mate better, it's important to have clean glasses," says the petite lady in charge. She looks like a kindly grandma. Someone is here selling flowers — which haven't been erotically arranged. Someone else is consulting on old-fashioned home decor. A couple hand out brochures advertising chalet rentals in the outlying Laurentian mountains. And two charming ladies extol the virtues of lipoidermy, a method of tightening skin and reducing tissue with a miraculous bandage doused in algae. Not exactly steamy. And what to make of a Laura Secord candy stall in a luvvv salon? What would Laura say? "She'd probably get a kick out of it, really," says the smiling student in the booth.

Where's the smut? Some of us have seen dirtier carpets. Sexologist Julie Pelletier has an explanation. "This is a very serious business," says the studious sexologist. "Sure, people need a little fantasy to put some spice in their love lives, but, ultimately, it's all about communication. And that's not necessarily sexual." It's clear that those who have come to the salon in search of cheap thrills will leave disappointed. "It's not bad, but it's not what I expected," says Manon, a single mother. "I'll just go home, make myself a plate of penis pasta, and go crazy." We think she's kidding.

It's two hours later, and Bobaru is still playing his Pan flute. "My love songs put people in the right mood," he says. "I can feel it." Yeah. But does Bobaru plop some Pan flute on the turntable when he makes love? "Not really. I get a little fed up with this music after a while. But, hey — it's a living." We think he's not kidding.

Wondering whether I'd been in some Pan-flute-induced trance and dreamed up everything, I return to the Salon de l'Amour et Séduction on another day. The good news is that my mind wasn't playing tricks on me. Again, I'm greeted by a potpourri of salespeople shilling romantic vacations, tastefully erotic photo sessions, baubles, massages, and . . . watches? Okay, Jean-Pierre, why watches? "Oh, watches can be very erotic," he replies. "You can time your erections and orgasms." This causes me to stammer, "But, but, wouldn't that distract one from the business at hand?" Jean-Pierre smiles, "Only the less agile."

I need help once again. Monique Lapointe is only too willing to oblige. She has to sit in her salon stall all day, anyway. She's been a sexologist for the last ten years, and business is booming. Monique has a theory: People are lonelier than ever, because they are held hostage by their careers. "But women are more open than ever about their sexuality," she asserts. That's good, right? Well, it depends on the gender. "The result of women being more liberated than ever is men being more terrified than ever," she explains. "They're worried about their sexual performance, about being judged, about being ridiculed. That's why impotence is on the rise." Bad pun, perhaps, but Monique has a point. Her theory does, however, go a long way towards explaining why Lorissa the Love Doll was selling like hotcakes at Vegas. No commitment. No snide remarks.

Monique acknowledges that there is a correlation between increased sales of sex toys and increased impotence. The same factors explain the proliferation of porno films, Internet fantasy chat rooms, and sex hotlines. "Many men today can do just fine with virtual people. It's the real people that cause them headaches and sexual problems," she insists. "The world has become a giant sex supermarket." Monique counsels her clients to screen erotica with their significant others as a means of overcoming dysfunction. "I'm talking romantic erotica, not hardcore porno," she says. "When patients, particularly men, watch hardcore porno, they start feeling inadequate again. They feel like they are failures unless they can perform the way the studs in the films do. Worse, they start to treat women as objects and not as equals." Monique isn't surprised by the stunning growth of the sex biz. "It goes hand-in-hand with the increasing sense of solitude most people find themselves experiencing today. Yet people want to satisfy themselves, so they will turn to whatever turns them on. But no matter how high-tech this business becomes, people will always need people to satisfy their innermost cravings for affection." It could be a long time coming for some. Monique fears the worst for today's young and restless. "They're Teflon kids." She shakes her head. "They're almost robot-like. They show next to no emotions. They're terrified of attachments, even with members of their families. It's frightening."

Chocolate penises and breasts and buttocks can also be frightening. And tasteless, according to one young man, who has just chomped down on a chocolate-covered butt sucker. They're being showcased on one side of the stall next to Monique's. On the other side, some teenaged girls are extolling the virtues of a potato-bug-like massaging critter, which is evidently all the rage for eliminating stress. What are the erotic implications, at least one curious mind inquires? Okay, it was me. "I wouldn't know, sir," replies Michelle, one of the girls in the booth. "This is strictly for relaxation purposes."

At the adjoining *Erospheres* magazine booth, Sarah looks about as relaxed as possible for someone wearing next to no clothing and trying to avoid getting doused with mustard by a passerby chowing down on a hot dog. A couple of well-placed straps and thongs are all that protect her from the elements and the voyeurs. Curiously, Sarah, twenty-six, is a clothing designer. She is married and the mother of two young children. She can also be seen in an issue of *Erosphere* striking a variety of suggestive poses, including one in which she performs fellatio on a young man unable to contain his enthusiasm. "Oh, that's my husband," she says, ever so demurely. "This modeling was a first for him, as well as me." Sarah signs her autograph on the spread for an appreciative customer. "I saw an ad in the newspaper asking for pretty women to send in their photos. So I did. And the next thing I know, I'm posing naked for everyone to see. I'm not shy." Clearly. "And I have nothing to be ashamed about." Clearly not. "I think I could serve as an example to other young mothers that posing naked doesn't end after having a couple of kids." Clearly. "Look, all I'm really doing is helping other people realize their fantasies. This is no crime, right?" Clearly not.

And then Bill Margold's words of wisdom jump back into my head once again. I ask Sarah, "What if your kids come home from school one day clutching a magazine with photos of you celebrating your sexuality with a candle up your butt?" Sarah doesn't even flinch. "Frankly, I'd be much more concerned if my kids had to come home from school to find a frustrated mother who couldn't express herself, rather than a mother who is proud of her body and sexuality. Okay?"

Annie Ouellet is fully clothed. A stylishly coiffed and attired mother of two, Annie, twenty-eight, could be a spunky account executive for some ad agency or a high-powered computer wonk. She doesn't look, let alone sound, like an editor of the province's biggest-selling skin mag, *Québec Érotique*. But she is. It's Annie's job to recruit models, set up photo sessions, and stimulate sales and readers. "I couldn't have dreamt of finding a more ideal job, either," says Annie, whose degree in communications has definitely come in handy. Confirming sexologist Monique Lapointe's thesis — to a point — Annie notes that women are becoming increasingly open about their desires. "They want more erotica in their lives, and it is my pleasure to help them attain their dreams." She flashes a big Welcome Wagon smile. Even Al Goldstein would be disarmed.

Annie introduces me to Quebec's biggest porn sensation, Cindy Cinnamon, star of the hot-selling vid *La Reine de l'Exhibitionnisme*. The flick is controversial, but not because Cindy does anything sinful with a goat, or anything. In fact, there are no sex acts per se in the entire flick. As the title implies, Cindy merely acts out her exhibitionist fantasies — by strolling naked down the quaint cobblestoned thoroughfares of her native Quebec City. What has invoked the ire of some city fathers — and what has consequently caused sales to go boffo — is the fact that real Quebec City firemen are seen gaping as Cindy demonstrates her prowess on a pole in a real Quebec City fire station. The curious firemen were suspended for a week without pay for standing idly by, and a star called Cindy was born.

"It was all an innocent mix-up," Cindy maintains. "We had permission from one level but not another." It was never Cindy's dream to become a fireperson, or even a film star. She wanted to become a vet. But she'll gladly settle for being the hottest porn star in the province. "I live very well as a result. I pay my taxes, because this business is entirely legal. Actually, I think of myself more as a cabaret performer along the lines of Lili St. Cyr." But Lili was likely never featured in a magazine photo spread stimulating herself with a gigantic metal rod. "It's really quite erotic, I feel," Cindy says. "There's no shame in that. I'm proud of what I do. My parents are proud, too. And my fans agree. Why else would little old ladies come up to me and just ask to hold my hand?" I give up. Why? "Because I am the sweet little girl next door who simply loves nature and animals." And who hates to dress — for any occasion.

Cindy says that she'd like to branch into comedy with a touch of sex. It shouldn't be much of a stretch. "Our role is to bring couples together," says Annie the editor. "There is no higher calling than that. The beauty of this business is that it's always reinventing itself and is never boring. Really, our work is primordial." Yet another word that you'll never hear from the mouth of Buttman. Along with Amsterdam, Montreal must be the most civilized sex capital in the galaxy.

"Sex is the most simple and beautiful form of expression mankind knows of," Annie continues, sounding much more like a pastor than a porno editor. But she has reason to be bullish. Her magazine even outsells *Playboy* and *Penthouse* in this province. "Sex is not just my work. It's my hobby. I'm giving people what they want and fulfilling my fantasies at the same time. I just wish the censors would understand that." The freethinking Annie does, of course, censure the selling of sex featuring animals or children. "That's not erotic. That's disgusting. At least doing what I do I can look at myself in the mirror every day and be proud."

There is a dancing penis on display at another stall. Its creator, too, seems awfully proud. Her name is Chantal Brault, and she is a practicing *néosexopédienne* — which only sounds like an occupation for which you could be arrested. There is no English translation for it. Brault's comely young assistant, yet another Annie, explains that it means a sexual healer or therapist. Annie is a devout follower of both Chantal's teachings and the dancing penises. "I was born to teach others about sex," claims Annie, twenty-one, who appears about as experienced as Anne of Green Gables. Nonetheless, she picks up a rotating, foot-long penis with purpose and describes how this object can give pleasure to both genders. "The beauty of this business is that you can't be easily shocked when you sell this sort of accessory," Annie tells me. "On the other hand, it doesn't necessarily suggest that because I sell this big rotating penis I have to use it." Chantal is now busy selling chocolates. Erotic chocolates. Annie states that chocolate can be very sensual, particularly when melted and smeared over a loved one. "It can be quite creative, too," she says. "A person can make artistic designs in chocolate on the body of a lover and then lick it all off. It's a great sensation and quite tasty, especially if it's Belgian chocolate."

André and Nicole are listening to this spiel. They are grandparents, but they are also quite curious. "This brings me back to my youth," André says. Comments Nicole, "There is no age limit for sex. Nothing shocks me here. We can talk more about sex today than we could when we were growing up, but there's still more progress to be made. Sex is the most beautiful thing in the world you can do for free." André and Nicole have retired, but only from their day jobs. He used to work as a taxman for the federal government. She was a nurse. She wears a little heart stamp on her cheek every day. "I wear my heart where the world can see it," she says. "When you hide your heart, life is over."

Sheryl Underwood doesn't hide anything. She bares her heart and her soul. She also throws out a whack of words you don't normally hear from women, especially on a stage. "I'm here to encourage every woman out there to suck a little more dick," Underwood, purse safely tucked under her arm, hollers into the mike. "Lick on that spot between the asshole and the balls! Y'all hear what I'm saying? There are rewards to be had." Lou Paget, watch your back. Sheryl Underwood wants to steal some of your thunder with a few tips of her own on the fine art of fellatio. The ladies in the house are hooting and loving every minute of it.

What gives? Well, something weird, perhaps even wonderful, has been happening the last few Julys at a Montreal nightclub. And it's something quite risqué, by civilized Montreal standards. Ladies — single, married, and pregnant — have been lining up to catch the extremely rude comedy stylings of our old pal Bobby Slayton and his handpicked coterie of reprobate cutups, mostly Yanks. It's all a part of the Montreal Just for Laughs Festival *Nasty Show* series.

Underwood, who has few peers, male or female, when it comes to spewing filth, is a *Nasty Show* highlight. After dispensing her advice to the girls, she has some pointers for the boys in the room: "If ya want your women to suck your dicks, then wash your nuts, ya nasty bastards." Again, the ladies in the room rise for a quick standing-O. "And guys," Underwood continues, "it wouldn't hurt if you learned to eat pussy. Don't be spitting in the pussy, okay? Cause we don't want to be getting gingivitis down there. And another thing, guys, don't pull your pants down too much, 'cause you ain't staying that long. We just want to fuck some of you, that's all. And, another thing, don't be just rammin' your dicks, 'cause we don't much like that, either." Another ovation.

Laughter is an irrational thing. There is certainly no logical explanation for the enduring popularity of *The Nasty Show*, but you can't argue with a convulsing audience. What started twelve years ago as a boys' night out has mushroomed into an event that draws as many women as men. In the early days, organizers were hard-pressed to fill Montreal's Club Soda for just two *Nasty Shows*. Now, there are a dozen shows, and tickets are as scarce as Bibles at Bobby Slayton's house. Over the years, Slayton, the abrasive Los Angeles comic, has become synonymous with this series. He does with dirty words what Picasso did with disjointed people on canvas. He makes art. And he makes audiences erupt.

What's most noteworthy about Slayton's legion of ladies is that they prefer to show up without their men. Times change. As mentioned, in years gone by, *The Nasty Show* was primarily a male preserve. Women showed up at their own risk. This is not to suggest that pit bull Slayton has turned poodle. Hardly — he's as raunchy as ever, as are his featured guests. No, it's more an indication of changing taboos, a reaction to the repressive attitudes that righteous agents of the moral authority have perpetrated for years to keep us in line. If nothing else, Slayton has succeeded in lowering the bar.

What might also endear Slayton to the ladies is the recent revelation that he's pro choice. "That's right," he screeches. "You can fuck me! Or you can blow me!" And, according to his world view, premature ejaculation is not a problem. Quite the contrary, in fact. "I beat you. I won." And he's sensitive. Sort of. "Feminists say strip clubs degrade women. Who's degraded? I walk out alone at four in the morning with a hard-on and no money." And he has more than a passing interest in evolution: "Who was the maddest dinosaur of all? T-rex! Small hands. Could never reach his cock."

In fact, *The Nasty Show* is most educational. Listen to the comics. Jackie Flynn, a wry Bostonian, makes this scientific observation: "The sperm bank is offering one hundred dollars a sample. Hell, then I've got a gym sock that's got to be worth ten thousand dollars." Flynn also comes clean about his orientation: "I'm not gay, but I think my hand is. I can't keep it off my dick." *Nasty*-circuit regular Jimmy Shubert, as well, has some fascinating theories about the differences between the sexes. His observations particularly delight the ladies: "Women might be able to fake orgasms. But men can fake whole relationships." Another Boston wit, Lenny Clarke, takes a dim view of Bill Clinton's dalliance with Monica Lewinsky: "He lied. A man might forget where he parks or where he lives, but he never forgets a blowjob — no matter how bad it was." Steve Marmel sees it this way: "I don't care if Clinton was fucking around. I don't even care if he was fucking around with my girlfriend. He was good for the economy. I can't get another economy."

Again and again, the biggest howls in the house emanate from the ladies. "I've been coming for years to this show, and

I can't imagine finding anything more entertaining," says a suburban housewife named Julie following one *Nasty* set. "The others can have their rock stars as idols, but I think I'm falling in love with Bobby. And, no, he didn't make me blush once. The point is that some men assume we can't handle that kind of raunch, but what kind of jokes do you think we toss around when it's only the girls?" Vicky, another *Nasty Show* vet, concurs. Her only concern is that by laughing too hard she might induce the birth of her baby, which is due in a week. "I'm sure even the baby got a kick out of it all. What a blast!"

The next set starts. A burly fellow, whom one is probably better off not messing with, is affronted by Slayton's bad taste. Meanwhile, the suburban moms are reveling in his shtick about specula and sperm. Interesting times we live in. The burly dude sprays some beer in Slayton's direction after the comedian directs a few choice comments his way. Springing to Slayton's defense are, of course, women. "The guy should really lighten up," says June, a fashion model and thirtysomething mother of two. "Men and women are so different, and it's fascinating to get Slayton's perspective on sex and relationships. What was that guy expecting? It's *The Nasty*, not *The Nice, Show.*"

You want insights into sexual politics and relationships? Call Germaine Greer. You want filth? You're home, honey. According to Slayton, men only have two feelings: "Horny and hungry." Not surprisingly, he gets grief from his wife for his Neanderthal views. "She always complains that I never talk to her after sex. I tell her that I talk to her before sex. In fact, that's why I talk to her." Pause. "Ah, you get married and your car insurance goes down, but she won't," Slayton laments.

Next, a former *Saturday Night Live* trouper, the unwell Dave Attell, touches a nerve in the female members of the audience when he admits that life on the road is lonely. "So I watch porno movies every now and again, and again and again . . . I've got a black belt in masturbation. I'm the Jean-Claude Van Hand in the field." Still, Attell balks at having sex with cows. "A horse, on the other hand, I could have sex with, because I'd always have a ride home."

Ever sensitive to the demands of his audience — the women want nasty women — Slayton has conscripted another funny lady, Carol Montgomery, for this set, and, like Sheryl Underwood, she proves that women can be almost as wicked as men. Fed up with men's complaints about having oral sex with women, Montgomery turns the tables: "You know, what men emit doesn't exactly taste like protein, as they would have us believe. It tastes like Clorox. Put it this way: if it did taste like chocolate, we'd have a game show." Nick DiPaolo then slays the ladies with his take on morality in Montreal. "You name a street after a saint that is mostly filled with peep shows. What? Is Saint Catherine the patron saint of chlamydia?"

Truth is, tawdry comedy is tough to do. There's a fine line between flatulent and funny. Any bozo can do shock toilet shtick. Some even make short careers in the field — hello, Andrew Dice Clay! But it takes a special talent to elevate filth to an art form. Slayton and frequent collaborator Robert Schimmel could well be the two best nasty men in the business. Their success is not accidental. Unlike Clay who was shrill, hateful, and, worst of all, humorless, Slayton and Schimmel mine the most intimate aspects of human sexual relations and bring a certain soulfulness to their subject matter. The material is disgusting all right, but darned if it doesn't crack people up. Timing and delivery are important, but mostly it's a matter of the boys making themselves the butts of their own ribald jokes. It really shouldn't come as a surprise that their cheeky stylings — essentially derived from the burlesque comedians of yore — strike a chord with women as well as men.

Schimmel can tackle the most squeamish subjects, but because he's so smooth and soft-spoken, he is able to disarm his audience: "It's not right to have sex with your pets, especially if it's a parrot. They'll tell on you to your friends." And Schimmel sounds positively Seinfeldian during this bit about inflatable love dolls. "Sure, she never has a headache, but you do after you blow her up." Slayton, who sounds like so much helium leaking out of a hot-air balloon, has some scruples, too, damn it! For example, he frowns upon the ménage à trois, "because that's *two* people you've got to talk to later." It's not all about sexual dysfunction, either. Over and over, Slayton proves that he is also a deep thinker: "How much do you have to hate your wife to ice fish in a frozen hole at five in the morning?"

Montreal is famous for many things. Of course, there's the food: bagels, smoked meat, poutine (a delicacy consisting of french fries, gravy, and cheese curds all melted together to form a congealed mass that could block the healthiest artery). Then there are the women. Panels of unbiased experts — okay, members of professional hockey and baseball teams as well as ne'er-do-well Hollywood actors and, of course, Slayton and his nasty boys — have deemed Montreal's women to be the very finest on the planet, at least the part of the planet they have visited, which is often Pittsburgh. Regardless, it is difficult to dispute this fact. In most of the world's major metropolises, spring is marked by flowers in bloom. In Montreal, spring is the time of year when men await with bated breath for women to shed their winter garments and parade around the city in skimpy yet chic attire. It's a ritual akin to the running of the bulls in Pamplona, except in this instance the onlookers pray to get butted by one of these babes.

Some of the city's pulchritude corps toil in the erotic dance trade. Catholic though Montreal may be on many levels, it has to have more strip clubs per capita than any other city in the solar system. Montreal is also considered to be the lap-dance capital of the solar system. That might have something to do with the fact that as of December 1999, lap dancing is no longer considered illegal or indecent — and there is a distinction here. One without the other could still land you in the jug. But there are constraints as to what constitutes legal and decent lap dancing. Not that the forces of decency and justice are faithfully monitoring the situation at all times, but contact must take place in a semiprivate cubicle in a strip club. The touching of a client's genitals is verboten. In fact, the lap dancer is supposed to stand with her hands on the wall of the cubicle while she is simulating nasty rituals. In keeping with Montreal's Gallic flavor, the lap dance is also referred to as "danse à dix," or ten-dollar dance — the price per tune for this type of performance art.

Now that we have established what the lap-dancing ground rules are, we can move on to matters of great cultural significance, such as the activities of The Killer Bees, a distinguished group of Montreal professionals. The Bees seek to expand their cultural horizons by touring the museums of the city and its environs, but at the museums they choose to frequent, nary a Picasso or a Monet is to be found. Certified Bee F.S., a prominent lawyer, equates this museum cruising with a search for the next *Mona Lisa*. But what he and fellow barrister Testy, along with the renowned Dr. Fred, mean when they say "museum" is actually "strip club."

Thursdays, The Killer Bees take their customary ringside table at Wanda's, an upscale downtown-Montreal strip club where patrons come to revel in artistry, not lap dancing. On this particular Thursday evening, the lithe and astonishing Tanya, resplendent in a leopard-skin bikini, is doing push-ups on the stage. Not that anyone doubted her fitness. Off comes the top, and Dr. Fred shakes his head. "Artificial tits," he proclaims. "I can always tell when they're artificial. The tits don't move. Also, a keen eye will observe that there is something a little off about the separation of the breasts." The astonishing Tanya also loses points with Testy when she tells him his cigar is stinky. Then F.S. tells Tanya that she'd never make it in Amsterdam, where cigars are not only enjoyed by strip-club customers but are also used by some of the performers; with their toned pelvic muscles, they light and smoke stogies through an orifice more commonly employed for the purpose of sexual reproduction.

The banter is all amicable. To her credit, the astonishing Tanya can strip and gyrate while denying to F.S. that she is carrying a load of ball bearings in her breasts. "Not at all," she protests. "I'm a vegetarian and I do yoga. I don't need implants." Dr. Fred isn't biting. The two engage in a discussion about the search for inner peace. The astonishing Tanya finishes her three-dance set and is replaced by the congenial Genevieve. The congenial Genevieve's best features — not to disparage her other ones — are her smile and near-perfect teeth. It works for F.S. He gives her a five out of five. Dr. Fred is in a funk. "They're fake," he shrugs. He is, naturally, referring to the congenial Genevieve's breasts. "Check out the flatness of her breastbone." Testy feels that Dr. Fred is being far too clinical: "You're taking all the romance out of it. If you have nothing nice to say . . ." Dr. Fred mutters, "Very well. She obviously works out." Genevieve, listening intently to the conversation, quickly adds, "And I'm into yoga, too."

In fairness, both the congenial Genevieve and the astonishing Tanya are excellent dancers. But it ain't their dancing that's brought them into this biz. So what is the congenial Genevieve's motivation? "In a word," she says, "money." The astonishing Tanya joins us. "Money is my motivation, too," she announces. "But I'm also an exhibitionist, and what other job affords me this sort of opportunity?" Tanya's hubby, a car salesman, didn't share her enthusiasm for exhibitionism. They recently split up. "My fantasies are my life," Tanya says. She also has a lucrative day job in the no-nonsense, non-exhibitionist field of nutrition — vegetarian nutrition. "That's why I still look great," she says. Although she could pass for twenty-five, Tanya turns out to be thirty-seven. She has a fourteen-year-old daughter. She has also been jiggling her booty, when not dispensing broccoli, for the last nineteen years.

Genevieve is getting restless. She is paid to dance on tables, not schmooze at them. Such is the role of the private dancer. "Time is money," she declares. "I'm out of here." But not before she collects some cash from The Killer Bees for the privilege of having her to talk to. Genevieve does allow, however, that she has had breast implants, but it was before she became a stripper. She also allows that she is not long for this business. She and her boyfriend are contemplating kids and a regular life. "I'm only twenty-four. That's plenty of time to start another life." The suddenly loquacious Genevieve concludes, "What we do here is sell fantasy. It's all aboveboard." Counters Tanya, "And we would never do porno films, no matter how much money they threw our way."

The girls aren't wanting for cash. They estimate that they each make two to three thousand dollars a week, depending on the demand for private table dancing. Tanya says that she invests a lot of her salary in accessories; flimsy though they may be, negligees and lingerie can cost plenty. "Customers don't want to see us in the same outfit night after night. We have to change or they'll get bored with us." Between her dancing and her day job, Tanya is pulling in close to two hundred thousand a year. "That sort of financial independence enabled me to leave my mate when he tried to control my life," she says. "He didn't understand that I needed to fulfill myself both as a nutritionist and as a dancer. But I'm also working as a therapist here. People come to complain about their wives, so I give them fantasy, but it's not like they want me to touch them or they want to touch me. They come simply to admire me. Dancers who let strangers touch them have no self-esteem." At ninety-five dollars an hour for table dancing, Tanya can afford to keep her self-esteem intact. Claims Tanya: "I think my customers would prefer it if I taught them how to breathe properly more than dance in their laps." Now I think you're pushing it a bit, Tanya.

Dr. Fred is having none of this. Although Tanya keeps insisting her breasts are real, he's unconvinced. "Those are surgical marks, I'm sure," he tells Testy. Testy replies, "You're taking all the romance out of this. We might have to excommunicate you from The Killer Bees." Dr. Fred is oblivious to the threat. "You want to see real breasts, check out Baby Honda's. Now those were mammaries." Baby Honda, according to legend and/or Dr. Fred, was a 350-pound stripper who worked in the boonies outside of Montreal. Her claim to fame was her ability to keep a roll of paper towels under each breast while she performed exotic acts onstage. "The enormity of her breasts — and they were enormous and they were real — allowed her to perform this feat," Dr. Fred marvels.

Tanya is not impressed. She is set to walk out on this discussion, but not before demanding one hundred dollars. "Time is money," she says. "You want to watch me dance? You want to talk? Doesn't matter. It's going to cost the same." But what about all this inner peace and yoga and broccoli, F.S. wants to know. "Vegetables aren't free," Tanya says. "I wish they were." Methinks there is an analogy here somewhere, but vodka has clouded my judgment.

I exit with The Killer Bees. We repair to a nearby joint for burgers, and The Bees plan the rest of the evening's merriment. After many burgers and much more liquid sustenance, they settle on Club Downtown, located right next door to the burger joint. A big sign on the door stipulates "legal contact," the buzzword for lap dancing and definitely not an invitation to mess with Club Downtown's humongous and currently mellow doorman, Mario. No sooner are The Killer Bees seated and checking out the onstage action than Dr. Fred offers a medical opinion. "Granted, they're only the size of cupcakes, but those breasts are real, damn it. They aren't rocks. They're much prettier." He's gazing at the nubile stripper before him. Testy acknowledges the authenticity of the breasts, but he is not blown away: "She can't dance. She has no moves. She has no talent."

Another dancer, wearing a hood that covers her eyes, takes to the stage and manipulates her cheeks rhythmically to the disco music. "Now that's a talent," Testy gushes. "Bravo!" The dancer gets a standing ovation for her butt movements, but the hood still covers her eyes. Dr. Fred also gives the blindfolded dancer a passing mark. Real breasts, too. He moralizes, "And she can lick them, which just goes to show there is no need to do harm to your body by getting implants when nature can take care of it." The next dancer lies on her stomach and spanks herself every thirty seconds. For the life of him, F.S. can't understand the point of this exercise, and he makes his displeasure known: "She doesn't have an ounce of talent or rhythm. Where is the pride?"

A patron at an adjacent table explains to Testy that legal contact means the dancers can't touch the customer, but the customer can touch the dancers — and the dancers will allow it, provided there is enough of a cash incentive. The price is negotiable. The patron's buddies emerge from a room at the other end of the club, where they have just forked over a small fortune, about five hundred dollars between them, for the pleasure of having a dancer in their faces — and then some. "I'd do it all over again," says one of these fellows, a college student from Boston. "I think I'm in love. I really feel that we had a connection. I think she liked me, too. Next time I'm sure she'll give me her phone number." Testy and F.S. merely frown. Dr. Fred, of course, wants to know if the college kid noted any surgical marks on the dancer's breasts.

The Killer Bees decide to split. "Is it a function of age when I enjoy the burgers more than the babes?" Testy asks. "I'm starting to worry about myself." But Mario the doorman is not plagued with self-doubt. As a gang of thirteen high-spirited young men meander in, Mario tells Testy that poor conduct is rarely a problem at Club Downtown. Nor can he recall the last time that some punk got fresh with a performer. "You don't have to worry about taking thirteen guys on," explains the doorman. "You just concern yourself with the biggest guy in the bunch. Once you deal with him, the rest are like little puppies and will do whatever you tell them."

Long after The Killer Bees have hit the sheets, twentysomethings James and J.D. hit the strip joints. Their hormones are constantly jangled. But because they are young and wealthy and unattached, they can afford to indulge their fantasies, which is precisely what they do every night. Some folks fly-fish for fun. James and J.D. "sport-fuck" for kicks. They also kickbox and race motorcycles, they are quick to add. James, with his Caesar-style bleached-blonde hair, believes that Montreal has become the world's sex mecca. "The women are beautiful and plentiful, and the price is right," he maintains, over a double Stolie on ice. "Two hundred bucks can go an awful long way in this town. Go to the Chicken Ranch in Vegas, and it will cost close to a thousand dollars, but the quality just isn't the same as here."

James runs a successful health food company, and he wants me to understand that he can get any kind of action he wants for free, but he prefers to pay for it, because then there are no strings; and, there's no limit to the thrills he can negotiate with a pro. In any case, he doesn't like to boast, but he's never met a nonpro who could keep up — or down — with him.

Tonight, James and J.D. have decisions to make. Do they travel to the small community of St. Jean, south of the city, for a tour of the clubs where anything goes? Do they go north to visit the clubs of Ste. Sophie, where almost anything goes? Do they head for uptown Montreal and hit Solid Gold? Do they stay downtown at Wanda's? Do they call up one of their favorite escort services? Or do they simply go to a massage parlor for an "R&T"? That's "a rub and a tug," in case you didn't know. Decisions, decisions. A rub and a tug sounds good to James, but at which outlet? He and J.D. estimate that there are a dozen massage parlors in downtown Montreal alone that offer this invigorating antidote to a day of stress. But J.D., a clothing manufacturer, would also like to have a few drinks. Which rules out the massage parlors as well as a certain haunt of theirs in St. Jean, which might be a bordello posing as a strip joint but which doesn't have a liquor license. So it's off to Wanda's they go. I tag along.

Sitting at the bar, James virtually ignores the dancers. He recalls J.D.'s recent birthday. What do you get for the guy who's got everything? James thought this over and came up with the idea of blindfolding his buddy and dragging him off to a motel. There, a hooker had her way with J.D. and vice versa. Unbeknownst to J.D., this birthday session was videotaped and copies were passed around to all of their friends. Overcoming his initial surprise, J.D. decided that he was pleased with his own performance and gave himself a thumbs-up. "If you think that's wild," he says, "you ought to see our Super Bowl party halftime shows." Evidently, the boys arrange their own entertainment in the form of several nubile dancers. "After the girls perform solo and together, the fun then becomes interactive," explains James. "Often, this stuff beats the football game itself." No doubt.

Party boy James is currently planning his brother's stag party. On hand for the occasion will be a bus, a few dancers, a couple of hookers, as well as friends and family members. After tooling around in the bus for several frivolous hours, they'll direct the driver to take them to a spot on the banks of the St. Lawrence River, where they will take in the Montreal Grand Prix. "Does James know how to throw a party, or what?" enthuses J.D. James takes his pal's admiration in stride.

Yet James insists that in the company of his new girlfriend he's a (slightly) different person. "Maybe she'd understand, but I think it's probably for the best that I don't tell her that I pay fifty dollars for a blowjob. It doesn't mean I like her any less. But I just see this as an extension of a massage to relieve all my stress. Even if I was married, I'd still go for my R&T." James allows that one day he, too, might settle down and get married. He may even have kids. "But why would I possibly want to do this now, when I have money and toys and so many choices of women?" He insists that the fundamental difference between himself and J.D. is that he doesn't quibble over the price of his pleasures. "J.D. is always bargaining," says James. "Sometimes I think he's more interested in the deal itself than the actual sex. Once, I recall, he was so pleased after getting laid for twenty dollars." J.D. doesn't deny any of this. He simply smiles.

James and J.D. feel, just a little, for the sucker who walks into a strip club, tells a dancer his sorry life story, and then actually believes he's won the lady's heart. "We call these guys patients or victims," J.D. explains. "They talk away to the dancer at the table and don't realize the dancer is charging them by the song, even if she is only talking." Standing next to the boys at the bar is the leggy Victoria, stripper/accountant/designer. Victoria doesn't disagree with J.D.'s assessment. She insists that she's heard enough tortured histories from her customers to enable her to add another slash to her job description: psychologist.

Even if James and J.D. were "patients," Victoria wouldn't be treating them tonight. The boys have decided to bolt Wanda's and head north to Ste. Sophie and Club C-Sexe-C. Half an hour later, we're there. The onstage action is your standard strip-club fare. James points to a section of private booths at the back of the club. "That's where the real action is. That's where you'll get the best lap dance in the province." The real action is also at the side of the stage, where the girls vigorously grope one another. Are they doing this to arouse the clientele? Not according to J.D. He believes that their years on the circuit have soured these women on men as sexual partners.

He tells the club deejay to play an instrumental version of "Hotel California" before he selects his private-booth companion. When I ask J.D. if he has a sentimental attachment to that particular tune, he replies, "Not at all. It just gives me more bang for my buck." The shrewd J.D. explains that the tune runs in excess of nine minutes. "Do the math," he says. "Most songs are three minutes long. This way my ten bucks goes three times farther, and it will take me only two songs to get off. I figure I'm saving twenty bucks." In a confessional mood, J.D. adds, "I'd rather get the girl to make out with me than anything else in the booth. That's the ultimate trip. But it's much more difficult." "Try dating, J.D." He rejects the suggestion. "It's not the same rush. This means getting a stranger to fall for you immediately. It's so sensual. It gets the blood flowing. And when we rub noses, there's no greater thrill." I'm confused: J.D. spends hundreds of dollars to satisfy his ultimate desire, rubbing noses with a stranger. "What can I say? Deep down, I'm really a romantic kind of guy."

While James is cavorting in a booth, J.D. figures he's found the right candidate for a nose rub. And so what if the deejay isn't spinning that nine-minute cut — J.D. can't wait. Four tunes later, he reemerges from a booth, along with a flame-haired dancer. He's all smiles. "She'll do anything, and I mean anything — suck, fuck, or even cluck — but she has got to get to know me a little better before she'll make out with me. I promised her I would come back and win her heart." Ah, young love — at ten bucks a tune.

Along the walls of this former bank, signs have been posted every few feet warning that sex is not permitted on the premises. Which would be understandable if the signs were funky holdovers from the days when the joint was a bank. Such, however, is not the case. These days, the building houses Club l'Orage International, Montreal's most renowned meeting place for swingers. And by swingers, I don't mean some breezy association of jazz beboppers. Nor am I referring to James and J.D., who would dearly love to swing but would find themselves unwelcome and lonely here — as would any single who ventured in. Members come, usually in couples, to meet other couples with whom they can exchange pleasantries, phone numbers, and perhaps even some carnal expressions. Sounds straightforward enough. But, oy — what headaches the owners of l'Orage have had to endure. In fact, the club's trio of owners should collaborate on a bluesy jazz number.

Club l'Orage International has to be the only wife-swapping club in existence where much of the decor consists of press clippings of the owners' legal troubles. It's no surprise that one of the three is a lawyer. Bernard Corbeil devotes an inordinate amount of his time, when he could be cuddling with other consenting adults, to contesting the law as it applies to

swinging. In July, 1999, co-owner Jean-Paul Labaye was convicted of running a common bawdy house out of his previous
base of operations, Club l'Orage, which had been in business
for three years at another location. Labaye has appealed the
ruling, contending that sex took place only among consenting
adults in the privacy of his apartment on the third floor of the
club. This apartment was not open to the public, and only
people (over the age of eighteen) who had been invited could
enter.

Regardless, Club l'Orage is gone, replaced by Club l'Orage
International. The establishment's third owner is the vivacious
Mapie. Corbeil, Labaye, and Mapie have vowed to stay on the
right side of the law by operating a meeting hall for swingers
where sex is not permitted and alcohol is not sold. To help get
the new club up and running, members pitched in. They reno-
vated the old bank building and decorated it with explicit etch-
ings of couples coupling and a few harnessed mannequins. The
three owners obtained a meeting-hall license from municipal
authorities and tried to establish the club not only as a rendezvous point for swappers but also as a venue for conferences on
sexual issues, erotic art displays, and intimate fashion shows. It
sounds simple enough. But the club was busted in April 2000,
not because lewd activities were taking place, but because alcohol was being served — albeit not sold — on the premises.
Corbeil and his partners were hopping mad. They believed that
club members had the right to bring their own booze. Not surprisingly, they felt that they were being unfairly targeted, and
they sued the Montreal police.

While Corbeil is less enraged these days, he's still somewhat frustrated. "They just don't understand what's going on
here," says the bearded, fifty-year-old barrister. "This is a European concept. Our philosophy is to be openminded and to be
respectful of other people's right to associate with whomever
they wish. This right of association is guaranteed in the Bill of
Rights." Revisiting these issues makes Corbeil's blood start to
boil all over again. He's sitting at the club's bar, once a line of

bank teller stations, and he's surrounded by a sea of legal briefs and press clippings and scrapbooks and seventy-five videos containing T.V.-news highlights, all relating to l'Orage's legal woes. "The Canadian Constitution guarantees the rights of people to collect stamps and butterflies and also to collect caresses. We have the right to be with people of common interest. Therefore, if we have the right to associate, then we have the right to have our own place."

Frankly, this legal stuff just ain't sexy. Given his druthers, Corbeil would be partying, not forever pleading his case. But he feels that there is a much bigger issue at stake here: basic civil liberties. And he'll go down fighting, if need be. To that end, Corbeil plans to recruit new members, and after he signs up the necessary number he'll issue each a sublease on the club. "Then, it will be a completely private place, where members will be free to do what they wish," he says. "This is for couples who like being with other like-minded couples, who like the idea of the nonexclusivity of sex. There are no laws being broken. But from the perspective of the police, they think swinging is disguised prostitution, which explains why just about all the other swingers' clubs around the city have been shut down. It's unbelievable. They have such puritanical ideas here."

Oddly, before the police raided l'Orage and the media storm erupted, most citizens of Montreal knew nothing about the swinger scene. The irony is that the busts have brought swingers the sort of recognition that money can rarely buy. Corbeil cites stats from a local newspaper survey in which sixty-three percent of respondents claimed to sympathize with the plight of swingers, supported their right to do what they wished in private, and chastised the local constabulary for over-reacting.

Jean-Paul Labaye saunters in, looking haggard. He has just missed his flight to his native France, where he was to visit an ailing parent. A chunky fellow with spiky dyed-blonde hair, Labaye lets Corbeil do the talking. And Corbeil has little difficulty in that domain. Labaye, he says, was on welfare in Montreal when he had the brainwave of starting a swingers' club. The original l'Orage was even endorsed by NASCA, the North American Swing Club Association, based in — where else — California. Though the name might conjure up wholesome images of barbershop quartets, Corbeil shatters the illusion. The association, he tells me, boasts a membership of more than forty thousand bona fide swingers.

Then Labaye pipes up, saying that the legal wrangling is beginning to wear him down. "It's reached the point where I'm making love to someone in my room and I hear a car speeding off on the street below, and I become distracted from the sex." This does not make Labaye happy. At forty, he's been swinging pretty much since he was physiologically able, which is to say for about twenty-five years. Although he's never married, he once had a relationship that lasted ten years — not to mention plenty of shorter ones. Jealousy has never been a problem for him or his mates, Labaye insists. "It's just a question of being open-minded and respecting others. I don't like baseball, but I defend the right of all those who do to go to baseball games." He won't even take a position on the thorny issue of whether swinging is preferable to monogamy. "It all depends on the person," he says. "It's obvious that for me swinging is more suitable for now. Who knows what the future might bring? Although I find it hard to imagine that I could live without it. On the other hand, though, I have advised couples I know not to swing, because it creates too much tension in their marriages. Like monogamy, swinging is not for everyone."

Joining Labaye at the bar is a fellow Parisian, Marie, who is on a short visit to Montreal. She's touching base with old chums. In her yellow ski jacket, Marie is the picture of innocence. She is also drop-dead gorgeous, with spectacular blue-moon eyes and an exquisite facial bone structure. She looks like French actress Sophie Marceau and could easily grace the cover of a fashion magazine. In fact, the twenty-five-year-old Marie is a lawyer. And she's a swinger — or she used to be.

Here's the kicker: as is the case with just about every swinger one may encounter at l'Orage, Marie swaps partners only when she is attached to someone. "When I had someone to swing with, I would swing," she explains. "But now that I'm no longer living with my boyfriend, I don't. The idea is to swing with the person you love, not simply as a means to get sexual gratification. It pleases me only to make love with someone else when my partner is around and doing the same. When you're comfortable with a person, you can share anything with them." This notion could prove shocking to nonswingers, who no doubt figure that swingers are essentially exhibitionist sleazoids looking to get laid at all costs. "That's a North American stereotype," Marie says. "In Europe, it's different. It's more accepted. There are many clubs, although I prefer the intimacy of just being with another couple at home."

Marie's friend Serge joins us at the bar. A trim, mustachioed Montrealer, Serge, forty-seven, has his own construction business. He and his partner, Carole, first met Marie and her then-mate Bruno at the original l'Orage a few years ago. The couples hit it off, and they started swinging with one another. Then Marie broke up with Bruno, and the swinging arrangement between the couples ceased — but most amicably. Now Serge and Marie are just buddies. And Serge says that Carole has not been up for swinging lately, mainly because she is still in mourning for her mother, who passed away recently. Like Marie, the congenial, straight-shooting Serge, father of two grown sons, insists that swinging is something you do as a couple, not as a single. Otherwise, you would be cheating on your spouse.

Evidently, an unconventional morality exists among these swingers. In a sense, they are more faithful to their partners than most other people are. It's somewhat akin to a set of Siamese twins getting together with another set to explore their shared interests. Marie doesn't refute this theory: "In many respects, we are so close to our partners that we are almost joined at the hip together." She cheerfully continues,

"Sex is an activity like any other that is more fun to do with others. I feel no taboo about it. It's not a question of being proud or not about what I do — it's just part of a lifestyle in which I'm comfortable." Labaye asks Marie and Serge if they plan to attend a fetish night at the club. Both decline. "Whips and leather don't really turn me on," says Marie demurely.

Mapie, the club's comely co-owner, struts over in a tight-fitting leather ensemble. A native of the Brittany region of France, Mapie, twenty-eight, says that she got into swinging five years ago. "It just happened. It wasn't something that me or my husband had planned," she says. "But now it's become part of our lives. It's something we share together." She also insists that it's something she would never do if her hubby wasn't present. Mapie, too, is of the opinion that swinging is not a panacea for all that ails a relationship: "If things are going badly, swinging can make it worse. But if they are going well, swinging can make it even better." Still, Mapie knows of a couple on the brink of splitting up whose marriage was salvaged by swinging. "They started at a nudist camp and then gradually got into swinging as the woman realized it was helping her fulfill needs that had been suppressed." Then the ever-philosophic Mapie offers the ultimate analogy: "Swinging is a lot like playing doubles tennis. Sure, it's quite a bit different from singles, but for those who are really into tennis, the two are both fun games."

Corbeil invites us into the club's more intimate lounge area, which turns out to be the bank's former vault. He explains the separate roles of l'Orage's co-owners: he is the brains, Labaye is the heart, and tennis aficionado Mapie is the soul. But all pitch in to perform the menial chores, such as washing glasses and cleaning ashtrays. "That way, we can see if people are fooling around too much, if you understand my meaning," Corbeil says. "If they are, we go up and tell them that we're part of the prolonged masturbation committee. The people will usually laugh, and stop what they're doing. They don't want to see us get busted by the cops again."

Talk of the cops gets Corbeil's dander up again. "The repression we've been dealing with is not unlike that experienced by religious groups and gays. It's like denying women the right to vote. We obey the rules. We don't allow minors in. There are no drugs and prostitution on the premises. We are not controlled by organized crime. And — oh yes — swingers have lower rates of divorce. So what exactly is the problem here?" Hard to say, but Corbeil would do well to seek the counsel of a few cops and judges. Evidently, there are several who are active members of his club. The plot thickens.

Sefi Amir lives a stone's throw from l'Orage. Although she is a broad-minded person who is sympathetic to her neighbors' plight, she has no interest in swinging herself. She is also preoccupied at present. Amir is a studious, bashful-looking artist with a cascade of Pre-Raphaelite curls. But when she's not adding to her ongoing series of paintings (renderings of haunting human faces) or attending art-school or stretching canvases for other artists (to earn rent money), the twentysomething, bespectacled Amir lets her imagination wander. Run wildly, in fact.

Amir has come up with a unique concept: a connect-the-dots drawing book. Such books are generally designed for children, but keep the young 'uns away from Amir's version. Dutifully connecting Amir's dots, would-be Picassos will likely be bowled over by the resulting sketches. The first of the eight connect-the-dot drawings the book contains depicts a rather intimate and erotic scene: a naked woman clutches the cheeks of another naked woman and eagerly licks her privates. I blush. On other pages, equally titillating sexual situations are revealed, featuring all manner of human couplings. I blush some more, but I am intrigued. My gosh, from the pens of innocent babes, such unabashed lasciviousness. The extraordinary thing about these dot puzzles is that the scenes they conceal are not at all obvious as one works at them. The images don't come into focus until the very last dots are connected. On the strength of this ingenious creation, we must welcome the unlikely Sefi Amir into the annals of illustrious porno pioneers.

Amir admits that the project was a bit of lark. She merely wanted to do a takeoff on the generic toy-store connect-the-dots book and create a little interactive fun, but she got carried away. Making the book was also a way for Amir to keep herself busy while her beau and room mate, Dylan Young, was deeply involved in his own artwork. In fact, it was through Young that Amir learned about porno in the first place. A studious and bashful-looking sort himself, Young has been consumed with creating an extensive series of rephotographs, using a technique favored by New York artist Richard Prince during the seventies. He takes photos of porno pics that he finds in magazines, on T.V., on video, or even on the Internet; he then reconfigures them by manipulating the color or the focus.

Like his lady, Young has a keen sense of humor. He's developed a game out of his series. He not only invites interaction among those who view his work, but he also affords them the opportunity of playing censor. Those who wish to participate are issued black dots, which they may stick anywhere on the photos. So, for example, if someone finds an ear offensive, he or she can simply dot it out. This enables the participant to concentrate on the sexual frolic depicted in the photo without distraction.

Both Young and Amir see their work as more than a clever novelty. They view what they do as a means of provoking people to address their personal sense of morality. "Sure, there has been an upswing in the acceptance of porn and new sexual attitudes of late, but there is still a backlash in some circles, even among the supposedly hip and liberated," Young opines. "Then again, some of the people who are into porno don't really understand it, either. They have been swept away by it all in a trendy way but without examining the issues at the root." And speaking of roots, Young shows me a recontextualized photo in which two well-endowed fellows enter a woman simultaneously from the front and the back. If the image jars the viewer, Young feels, then so much the better. "What I want to do is simply mirror society's reflection of porno."

It's work, sure, but Young confesses that it sometimes turns him on. Amir, too. "I guess my connect-the-dots idea was born from watching him work so painstakingly on his project," she says. "I have a similar confrontational approach, but I just have my own ideas on how to get that across. The drawing book is as liberating for me as it is for those who connect the dots." Amir went through her mate's research photos and images to find appropriate scenes for her book. She made line drawings from these and then reduced each drawing to a pattern of dots. Prior to hooking up with Young, Amir hadn't taken a position on porno, but she has since come to endorse it as a vital thera-peutic tool. "It's a market commodity, which, if it can titillate people at home to have enjoyable sex with one another, is a wonderful thing," she says. "And if it can earn artists and per-formers a living at the same time, it's an even more wonderful thing."

Young believes that porno is not so different from the kinds of entertainment and advertising that are currently being mar-keted to mainstream audiences: "We're already being sold dressed-down, watered-down titillation in T.V. soap operas, rock videos, and Calvin Klein ads. But the creators of this stuff are still skirting the issues. Why not address the subject head-on?" Amir concurs: "If the creators do that, it will simply mean better porno being made by young, hip artists. And fuck the narrative, let's just go for better images."

What concerns both artists most is censorship. "You have to ask what the watchdogs of morality are trying to protect us from," Young says. "Is it that they don't want people to know that there's more than one hole in which to enter a woman?" asks Amir. "Sure, some things repel me, so I just don't watch them." Reflects Young, "But I don't think adult porno encour-ages sexual victimization. It has more to do with society's inabil-ity to deal with its inhibitions and its unwillingness to accept or express sexuality." This gets Amir going: "It's such a joke. Some people think the women in the industry are being exploited. No one wants to hear that many are in it willingly, happily, primarily for the money. There is a huge hypocrisy at play. Some women's groups are forever trying to save prostitutes, but what they're doing is taking them away from their livelihoods. If they just legitimized the business, it would be better for all concerned."

And don't get Amir started on the popular notion that porno reduces women to stereotypes: "I think it's the opposite." So does Young: "There is a much wider variety of women's body types in porno than in regular Hollywood movies. You see women of all ages, shapes, colors, and backgrounds. It's more representative of the world around us. It's a much less homogenized view than what you see in everyday pop culture. Look at the fashion world. It's a very uniform construct." Young then refers to the writings of Havelock Ellis on the psychology of sex: "Women in countries accustomed to wearing no clothing had no sense of shame at all, until others from countries where women wear clothing told them it was wrong."

Young feels so comfortable in the company of naked women that he goes to strip clubs, not cafés or bars, to study or research. "What I like about the setting is that the women are completely in control." As for Amir, she is hoping that her mate will arrange to have a lap dancer perform for them at a club. "I just want to experience the same thrills he does. We are entirely faithful to one another, but I don't feel that it's cheating if we're just watching others perform. Movie dramas make you cry; pornos make you horny. It works for me." Young thinks it's just good, dirty fun. No more, no less. "The point is not to become obsessive," he says. "It's, like, being addicted to collecting baseball cards isn't healthy, either. We just have to put porno in perspective: it's simply an escape that can be quite entertaining and interactive." And, in the case of Amir and Young, quite profitable.

The big sex buzz in Montreal at present has nothing to do with swingers, fetish nights, lap dancers, or connect-the-dots. Would you believe that hairstyling is at the center of the commotion? Uh-huh. So what was the moral authority's first clue that Le Salon Sex Symbol, in the Montreal suburb of Laval, was offering more than rinses and razor cuts to its clientele? Evidently, the establishment's sign alone wasn't sufficient to alert the police. Nor was the fact that the salon had one room for cuts and three rooms furnished with sofas and VCRs that played porn vids.

After an exhaustive two-month investigation, the Laval constabulary finally deduced that the stylists at Le Salon Sex Symbol were also strippers. They danced dirty. They talked dirty. And, yes, they even managed to give the occasional trim, although it is believed that customers weren't flocking to the establishment for a good haircut. For five years, the salon had flourished, mostly because its "stylists" would bare their breasts for the customers, strip, touch, and engage in erotic shows — no small feat, the latter, while clutching clippers and a comb. As a consequence of their investigation, the Laval police arrested three female employees and five male patrons, who apparently did some dirty talking as they were being dragged away. They were charged for working in, or frequenting, a bawdy house.

Curiously, erotic hair salons are legal in the province of Quebec — if no touching takes place, that is. And there's the . . . um . . . rub. The law sees no problem with a stripping stylist, which is well and good. But the question that begs to be answered is this: How does a barber shear locks without touching her customer? The law is at a loss as to how to explain that one.

Le Salon Sex Symbol conducted a major advertising campaign a few months before it was busted. In spite of this, the police admitted that they only took action when they started receiving frantic phone calls from the wives and girlfriends of men who had been patronizing the place. These women complained that their significant others were offered an array of sexual services, and, worse, that they were not amused with the coiffures their men had received. After a couple of undercover police officers visited the salon and were propositioned by the stylists, they raided the joint. According to the police, a haircut from a flimsily attired female stylist at Le Salon Sex Symbol would set you back twenty-two dollars. But, for an extra ten dollars, the stylist would bare her breasts. For another ten dollars, she would remove all of her clothing while cutting your hair. An additional forty dollars would buy you an exotic show. And, for a mere thirty dollars more, the stylist would caress you. Oh yeah — ten additional dollars would get you a mouthful of seductive conversation. That works out to $122, tip not included.

Although they couldn't prove it, the police were convinced that some customers paid to have sex in the salon with their bountiful barbers. And what led the cops to believe that something off-color was taking place? Well, when the police raided Le Salon Sex Symbol, they happened to find the comely twenty-eight-year-old owner with a male client. The two were naked and fiddling with a vibrator, oils, and Kleenex. And no scissors were in sight. In fairness, however, police did concede that haircuts were occasionally performed at the salon. "We found some hair on the floor," one officer noted. "Apparently, they have a few clients who just go there for that."

With the stylists' shears temporarily out of commission at Le Salon Sex Symbol, some thrill-seekers have decided to hunt down the fabled Erotic Car Wash in east-end Montreal. This joint gives brand new meaning to a buff and a hosing. According to local legend, off-duty strippers go there to wash all manner of vehicle and, sometimes, their drivers, while wearing little clothing. I comb the area with our lap-dancing enthusiasts, James and J.D., and we ask the locals, but no one knows whether the car wash is still in business.

At one point, the owner, Mario Bellavance, who had also run seven fully clothed car washes around the city, had talked of selling Erotic Car Wash franchises across the province. But those were heady times for Bellavance. Drivers would pull into his two-car garage to watch as many as eight scantily clad women in very wet T-shirts tenderly wash their sedans. The charge was twelve dollars, and the entire operation took about ten minutes — depending, of course, on the lineups. Not only that, but also some customers were so taken with the experience that they would bring their vehicles back two or three times a night. In the early days, as many as 120 cars would be serviced nightly. So Bellavance, riding high, announced that he was hiring men to cater to the needs of female drivers. He already had thirty women on staff.

But it wasn't all smooth sailing for Bellavance. The neighbors complained. One woman was particularly peeved that her kids were forever trying to peep through the car wash's steamy windows. Undercover cops paid frequent visits to make sure that the staff was only hosing the cars. Bellavance responded by covering the windows and advising his employees to abide by a strict work code — that is, they were not to enter cars or have contact with drivers. Damn, no Armorall on the gearshifts. Furthermore, drivers under eighteen were forbidden to enter this kingdom of bubbles, and Bellavance began carding his clients.

So where did the Erotic Car Wash go? Area residents aren't sure, but the mythology of the place has grown. According to one fellow, there is now a floating erotic car wash. "They try to stay one step ahead of the law," he says. "There are no signs. The hours are irregular. Mostly, the action takes place between midnight and three in the morning, when the downtown strippers come off their shifts." But how can he be certain that it's still in operation? "Simple. When you see a car that is spotless, in the middle of the night, following a snowstorm in the city, you know something is up. And when you see a beautiful young woman walking around in frosted T-shirt when it's forty below zero, you don't have to be a Sherlock Holmes to realize she's been doing plenty of polishing." The fellow wants to give Bellavance his due, explaining that when a customer couldn't afford a car, the boss would simply lend him one to bring in for a wash. "The man was a hero in parts of the community." A real Robin Hood. Even if he left the hood work to others.

Chapter 7

Don't Ya Just Love This Frozen Tundra?

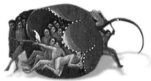

CANADA

The setting is the twenty-fifth annual Miss Nude Canada Pageant, in Winnipeg, Manitoba. Think Winnipeg, and chances are you're not thinking nude. Unless it's frostbitten. And then you surely don't want to think about it at all. Only our thrill-seekers James and J.D. do — but they think of nothing but nudes, all kinds, all the time. And so this particular pageant marks one of the highlights of their social season.

Mercifully, James and J.D. can remain indoors for this event. That's because some of Canada's most exquisite exotic dancers have also opted to avoid the frost throughout the pageant; they want to avoid exposing themselves to the hostile elements that can bedevil Winnipeg during the winter. The pageant's title is something of a misnomer in the sense that the competition is pretty much limited to Canadian professional strippers, as opposed to those Canadian nature-lovers who get their kicks romping through flora and fauna and bear droppings in the buff. In addition to James, J.D., and the beer-drinking gents in the audience, on hand to witness the contestants peel off their clothing while performing calisthenics around a pole on a no-frills stage is documentary director Paul Borghese.

The name of Borghese's latest oeuvre is *The Canadian Ballet*. This may conjure up images of little tykes in tutus tiptoeing their way through a Christmas rendering of *The Nutcracker*. Wrong idea. According to Borghese, "In Canada, there is an industry that is treated with more respect and credibility than it is in the U.S. or anywhere else in the world. In parts of the country, its members are required to be licensed as burlesque entertainers. However, devoted fans have given this exotic performance art form a name of their own, which truly reflects their high regard: The Canadian Ballet." Very moving, even if no Canadian I've ever met has heard the term before.

Tarnishing the rep of Canada's vibrant classical dance scene is clearly not Borghese's mission. In *The Canadian Ballet*, he encourages his subjects to bare all — their thoughts, anyway. And they do. Stripper after stripper concedes that the work is tough yet fun and lucrative, that she loves the applause and the attention, that she's a "real" person who goes home to husband and kids and, if time permits, does the laundry. Stop the presses.

Unless watching an Annie Oakley-type firing her six-guns onstage on her way to achieving total nudity turns your crank, *The Canadian Ballet* isn't exactly a turn-on. The interviewed dancers are so earnest, so open, so sensitive, so darned sweet, that you'll be struck by lightning if you should begin to harbor unholy thoughts about them. One of the dancers is a former classical ballerina. She spent sixteen years in a tutu waiting for the big break that never came, but she still yearned to perform. Stripping is dancing, after all. It's the bloody Canadian Ballet, right? And the money is pretty good, too.

But don't get the wrong idea. It's not all a romp in the bush. A stripper's earnings must be reinvested in catchy costumes, 'cause the Annie Oakley garb won't fly forever. Plus, there is the pressure to change routines regularly and the grueling hours of rehearsal. Some of Borghese's subjects talk about how they are constantly compelled to come up with new ideas. One stripper decides to dish out ice-cream cones while she flashes her . . . cones. Another figures that getting herself tricked out like Cleopatra is the ticket . . . yet another is stuck on Spider-woman. According to Annie Oakley, or perhaps it's Cleopatra, you just have to abide by the stripper philosophy. It's deceptively simple: "Look sexy. Be happy. Fulfill your fantasies. And get the guys on the side of the stage to clap." That's what it's all about.

Canuck strippers insist that they are poles apart from their counterparts to the south. "The Americans walk out in their Wal-Mart underwear and just jiggle," according to one of the dancers in Borghese's film. "They think audiences will go wild just by doing that. Well, you have to work your ass off to get ahead." One of her colleagues bristles at the mention of the movie *Showgirls*, which purports to blow the lid off the business: "Nobody I know does lap dancing like that in Canada. I wouldn't even do stuff like that in bed. We have a cleaner image here." To maintain it, Canadian strippers work out so that they can execute cartwheels and headstands. It's all part of what you have to do to earn a decent living. In fact, some of the strippers say the money is so good that they have been able to buy themselves fancy cars, homes, apartment buildings, and even businesses where they can work with their clothes on. Wonderful, but is there a downside? Why, yes. A few of the women suggest that not all racks are created equal. "Girls with big boobs do better." Thus, many feel they have no choice but to get their breasts enlarged. Also, their line of work isn't conducive to finding Prince Charming, or anyone at all who's charming. "We attract a lot of mooches, losers, drug dealers, or male dancers," one stripper laments. And this is before she encounters James or J.D.

Speaking of James and J.D., the pageant is over, and the boys are disheartened. It wasn't anything like what they'd expected. And the performers were all faithful to their fellows. To make matters even worse, in their downtime the boys have come upon a report in *The British Medical Journal* that confirms the biggest fear of at least half the human race. Drat! Male menopause, or manopause, does indeed exist — and we can't blame Maggie Thatcher, either (okay, maybe just a little). This condition apparently explains why so many middle-aged men suddenly saunter off to Amsterdam to study the banana up close or buy fancy sports cars they can't afford. They are actually suffering from a decline in male hormones; theirs is not unlike the plight of women, who run out of eggs in middle age. The symptoms, too, are similar: hot flashes, fatigue, insecurity, decreased sexual interest, and, of course, increased appetite for junk food and Oprah. These are just some of the findings (save for the one about Oprah) of Duncan Gould and Richard Petty of (and how's this for the best euphemism you've ever heard?) the WellMan Clinic in London.

Gould and Petty note that testosterone levels decline dramatically as men age, that by the time they hit the big 5-0, half the men in the world lack the sex drive most young men have early in the morning. All right, fuhgeddabout that morning roll in the hay. What happens at night? Well, it seems that with advancing age there is a breakdown that results in the lowering of testosterone levels by evening. This is all rather distressing, but the WellMan boys believe that they have a solution — one, incidentally, that has been stiffly criticized by other experts in the field. Gould and Petty propose a testosterone-replacement therapy that would treat manopause much the way hormone-replacement therapy treats menopause.

Now if all this sounds a tad too clinical for your tastes, you will certainly perk up when you hear about the more user-friendly advances in the field that have been achieved by Dr. Jeffrey Fuhr, a forward-thinking, fun-loving psychologist living in quaint, colonial Victoria, British Columbia (where, ironically, many of the inhabitants are aroused by Maggie Thatcher). So, it's off to see the Lizard Wizard in Victoria, considerably west

of Winnipeg, but a little shy of the Pacific Ocean, and still in
Canada. Fuhr just might have a cure for any libido woes you
may have that won't hurt a bit. In fact, it's quite tasty. All you
have to do is ingest a few of your favorite confections — chocolate, popcorn, peanut brittle — mixed with a handful of passion herbs, and poof! You're a stud once more.

Working out of an integrated Victoria health clinic, Fuhr
had at one time been specializing in men's health problems,
specifically those involving sexual inhibition, impotence, and
decreased sex drive, as they are related to male menopause.
"Most men over thirty-five go through intermittent periods
where they are impotent or mildly impotent, and they get extremely anxious about it," says Fuhr. "If a man can't get an
erection, he gets terribly worried about it. That's what makes
it an even worse problem than it really is." Fuhr had observed
that bound-up testosterone in muscles and tissues resulted in
men getting flabby and losing hair, not to mention sex drive.
He also noted that certain herbs could clear up the bound testosterone. He was particularly encouraged by the results that
the clinic's homeopaths and naturopaths had achieved with patients. So he began doing intense research in the area and discovered that there were an enormous number of Viagra-like
natural alternatives on the market. One herb kept cropping up:
avena sativa (that's green oats to you). Fanciers of this oat
claimed to have experienced radical improvement in sexual
prowess and earthshaking orgasms, among other things.

Then it came to Fuhr that there was a massive market out
there comprised of folks not only afflicted with sexual problems, but also with busy lives. And so Loving Foods was born.
Loving Foods is a company that mixes confections with herbs
containing aphrodisiacal properties. "I went this one step further because most antidotes to these problems are in pill form,
so they still have the connotation of medication and pseudo-
medication," Fuhr explains. And that's a turn-off. Fudge, on
the other hand, isn't. So Fuhr got out the food processor and

started fooling around with fudge and peanut brittle and herbs; he came up with something that approximated a tasty treat that just might make folks horny.

Fuhr tried his concoctions out on friends and neighbors. And guess what? They all reported that they were greatly stimulated in the boudoir. Fuhr was intrigued. "When I questioned them, they all told of different experiences," he says. "When people made wild claims about what had happened, it started to occur to me that this was as much due to their own expectations and fantasies as it was to their own individual responses to the herbs. Some people were telling me they had never felt so energized, that they never realized they could go for so long." Fuhr began organizing tasting parties. "When I would tell people what sort of things they might expect, they would then say they felt a tingling in certain areas or that they were feeling flushed. People started to giggle. There was a kind of contagion phenomenon. People just couldn't wait to get back home and start experimenting with their partner."

It occurred to the good doc that people's expectations might be even more potent than the actual properties of his chocolate-covered herbs — that, indeed, a lot of their sexual angst could be in their minds. Whatever. Fuhr decided to build in even more expectations by including kinky-ish instructions with the products. For example, his caramel concoction was accompanied by the suggestion that the consumer tear a strip off the product, wrap it around a finger and then have a lover lick it off. "What this does is to stimulate the intimacy between the consenting partners and to create a context for the herbs to work," Fuhr notes. Then he went even further. He decided to put no herbs at all into a Loving Foods bread mix and place the emphasis instead on the preparation. To wit: "Twenty minutes before your lover arrives, put on your apron — only your apron — and greet your lover at the door." Out of the view, one hopes, of nosy neighbors. Back to the instructions: "Act nonchalant as you take the bread out of the oven, and then offer your lover the first slice." Not only is this fraught with symbols, but it's also, Fuhr insists, a turn-on. "What I've discovered is that the actual amount of aphrodisiacs becomes almost less important to the context." This is all by way of saying that Loving Foods products don't work the same way for everyone. "Look, people have different metabolisms and constitutions," says Fuhr. "We're not making any therapeutic claims here. We're not saying this cures impotence."

If such a cure was all he wanted in an herb, Fuhr could have fiddled with the yohimbe, which is highly effective in dealing with erectile dysfunction. Fuhr explains that yohimbe works by irritating the lining of the genitals and will succeed in creating an erection. But at what cost? And how much fun would it be? Some scientists and doctors have expressed concerns about the longterm effects of Viagra and other such stimulants. Fuhr emphasizes that many of these remedies don't just work automatically; they have to have an arousal context. And that's where Loving Foods comes in. Reaction to his experiments has been so overwhelming that Fuhr has set up a Web site — www.lovingfood.com — to market his munchies.

He obviously takes as much pride in the naming of the products as he does in their accompanying instructions, their ingredients, and their healing powers: Possession Popcorn, Brazen Brittle, Funky Fudge, Ritual Chocolate. Consumers get aroused just pronouncing these names. And what to make of Fuhr's preserves: Red Pepper Thrust and Garlic Girl? Or his condiments: Mexican Lick and Makeout Mustard? On the other hand, what could be more fitting to spread over your hot dog? Fuhr offers a guarantee and a slogan with his products: "Consensual Treats for Lovers." To date, he hasn't had a single request for a refund from an unsatisfied customer. Fuhr also takes great pride in the relative merits of his various goods, all of which cost between eight and sixteen dollars each. Possession Popcorn, intended for new lovers, contains "heart-opening" herbs, like hawthorn and juniper, and no aphrodisiacs. Fuhr is particularly fond of the popcorn, because it is caramel-coated. "I have to admit I love it so much that I eat the stuff all the time," he says. Is he suggesting that he's perpetually aroused? "Let's just say that I have rarely been more energized," replies the doctor, who is single. "Even if someone discovers that the products don't arouse them, no one will ever be able to deny that they are at least quite scrumptious. But we truly feel we have found a niche in the market, a real growth area [pun almost certainly intended], and it's only a matter of time until these products are firmly established," states Fuhr. "At worst, I've got a whole basement full of chocolate." And at best he's created a loving, if chunky, planet.

Our odyssey into the wide world of sex, boys and girls, ends not with a bang, but with a thump — on the computer, at the other end of Canada, where the Atlantic Ocean comes into play. We're talking Internet here — the wacky, high-tech innovation that has allowed sex pioneers to go boldly where their ancestors never went. But first, a message from the church: a thousand Hail Marys for all you online pervs. If millions around the world can twig to the notion of virtual sex, then they should be able to grasp the concept that they are also committing a virtual sin. So says the renowned Roman Catholic magazine *Famiglia Cristiana* (Christian Family). Yup, if Moses were to descend and walk among us these days, he might well be inspired to add an Eleventh Commandment: Thou shalt not commit cyberlust.

Evidently, even flirting on the Net with someone other than your spouse has been deemed online adultery and a sin in the eyes of the church, according to *Famiglia Cristiana*. "Switching on your computer and exchanging confidences with people you have never met, to relieve the tedium and frustrations of a dull marriage, amounts to betrayal, even if your mistress or lover exists only in the ether," the Italian newspaper *Corriere della Sera* pronounced in commenting on the report. Reverend

Antonio Sciortino, the magazine's religious editor, places evil thoughts on the same sin plateau as evil deeds: "Those who log on with amorous intentions, either to look at erotic images or to talk to a virtual lover, must not kid themselves that surfing the Internet will wash their sins away. For Christians, there can be no moral difference between a virtual affair and a flesh-and-blood betrayal."

No surprise, then, that the Vatican, which has been bullish on the World Wide Web, is offering an online confession service to sinful surfers. This, in addition to trying to entice them into church chat rooms. But, according to a *London Times* report, the Vatican has warned that absolution still requires a face-to-face encounter between priest and parishioner. "The Devil is out there on the Net," says Franco Mastrolonardo, a parish priest at the forefront of the church-chat-line movement. This virtual brouhaha appears to be emanating from a survey published in *Il Giornale* that indicates one out of two Italian women is jealous of the time her husband spends at the computer. Many of these women deal with their jealousy in decisive ways. Thirty-six percent of respondents allowed that they have arranged for a steady stream of calls to tie up the phone line, while twenty-three percent conceded that they have buggered up the computer by pulling out plugs or tinkering with the software. A staggering forty percent confessed that they fear their hubbies will find new mates in cyberspace. *Il Giornale* suggested it would be more effective for wives to threaten their significant others with damnation and to remind them that Jesus can monitor all of their activities, even in a salacious Internet chat room.

This kind of tough talk might cut it with some virtual sinners, but not Eric Albert. For starters, he's not Roman Catholic. Even if this nonpracticing Jew were, it's doubtful that any Vatican edict would inhibit his Internet explorations. Albert is a prominent, middle-aged architect living in the hip burgh of Halifax, Nova Scotia. He rises early each day to jog through a scenic oceanside park. On weekends, he reads, plays squash, and goes on family outings with his second wife, Margo, a prominent film-documentary editor and a nonpracticing Presbyterian, and their six-year-old daughter, Chelsea, who just finished kindergarten at the local Montessori school. Albert has a twenty-one-year-old daughter, Grace, from his first marriage, who studies psychology in Chicago. Eric is forty-eight. Margo is thirty-nine. They have a healthy sex life — they indulge 2.3 times a week, as close as they can figure.

Eric is in a particularly festive mood this evening. He has just landed a lucrative deal to design a strip mall in the outskirts of Halifax. Although he prefers reconfiguring older homes for well-heeled clients, shopping centers pay the rent. To cap off this glorious day, Eric and Margo, unrepentant oenophiles, have broken out a prize 1991 Chateau Saransot-Dupré, a Listrac-Médoc, from the cellar of their dazzling, postmodern downtown digs. "Excellent nose," comments Eric as he takes a last sip. "A nice soupçon of leather and a fine hint of plum, too." Margo nods. Indeed, the wine has perfectly complemented the barbecued flank steak, the endive salad, and Margo's knockout potato salad, not to mention the Morbière and Chauvingnol chèvre that rounded out this repast. Eric, slightly giddy, grabs a relatively more pedestrian Merlot from Oregon, and we retreat to his study. It's nine P.M. Margo is putting Chelsea to bed. And Eric can now unwind by engaging in his fave nocturnal activity: fantasy. He fires up his fully frilled computer, signs on to America Online, and prepares to get randy by pretending he's someone else.

I watch as he takes on one of his many Internet alter egos: CindyCan18, which is code for eighteen-year-old Cindy from Canada. CindyCan18 has e-mail. Hi23maleBurbank would like to chat and, eventually, meet CindyCan18, at her convenience. CindyCan18 is also inundated with ads for custom-fit golf clubs, weight-loss pills, and get-rich-quick schemes, like Please Take our $10,000. Next, CindyCan18 clicks onto the Life network. She breezes by the twenty-three chat rooms for Christian Beliefs, the Fabulous Fifties, and Pagan Tea Houses, and goes straight to the New Young Adult quarters — or as CindyCan18 prefers to call it — the "Wut-up Room." CindyCan18 alerts other New Young Adults that she has just sashayed into the room and is ready to ruminate.

Estabon20 contacts her immediately: "Hi, CindyCan18." To which she responds: "Hi, Estabon20." Pouring himself another glass of wine, Eric muses, "This could be the beginning of a beautiful relationship."

Estabon20: "What up?" CindyCan18: "You mean 'what's up'? [Eric can't resist] Essentially, I'm a spelling dominatrix." Estabon20: "Yes, you're right." CindyCan18 is about to type, "What do you look like?" but she reflects and changes her mind. Says Eric, "No, I'm the girl here. I'll wait for him to tell me."

Estabon20: "How old are you?" CindyCan18: "Duh. It's like my handle says. 18." Eric murmurs, "I don't think Estabon20 is very bright." This impression is reinforced when Estabon20 fires back that he's not twenty as his monicker might indicate, but rather seventeen.

CindyCan18: "We almost the same age." Estabon20: "Yeah. What you like to talk about?" CindyCan18: "I dunno. U?" Estabon20: "I will like to talk about sex if u want." CindyCan18: "Sex?" Estabon20: "U a virgin?" CindyCan18: "No. Sorry. Does that make u mad?" Estabon20: "Oh no." CindyCan18: "Oh good." And so the mating process begins, much to Eric's amusement.

Estabon20: "How old was the guy you sleep with?" Cindy-Can18: "20." Estabon20: "20?" CindyCan18: "That's right." Estabon20: "That ok." CindyCan18: "Phew. I don't want to put you off."

As CindyCan18 conducts her private chat with Estabon20 on one side of the computer screen, EZToo sends a general message on the chat room's menu: "Any white chics in here into black guys?" CindyCan18 alerts EZToo that she's ready to rap. Meanwhile, Estabon20 is still on the scene: "Do you know what is cyber?" CindyCan18: "What is cyber?" Estabon20: "Don't get mad." CindyCan18: "I won't."

The ever-versatile CindyCan18 is now conducting two chats simultaneously. EZToo: "Ever been with a black dude?" Cindy-Can18: "No." EZToo: "Don't be embarresssed."

In another part of etherworld, Estabon20, who has had a long time to ponder CindyCan18's question about the true nature of cyber, replies: "Sex in the computer." Ever the inno-cent, CindyCan18 punches in: "How do you have sex in a com-puter?" Estabon20: "I tink that what it is."

EZToo drifts back: "Ever been with any guys?" CindyCan18: "Yes." EZToo: "You'll really like black guys." CindyCan18: "Why?" EZToo: "Were bigger." CindyCan18: "Bigger?" EZToo: "Bigger dicks!" CindyCan18: "Blush." EZToo: "We're very oral. You like giving or recieveing?" CindyCan18: "I like oral." EZToo: "Oooooh girl, I think I be fallin' in love."

Not wishing to alienate Estabon20, the dexterous Cindy-Can18 composes this for him: "Can u talk dirty?" Estabon20: "What are u waring?" CindyCan18: "Tank top. Shorts. It's very hot here now." Estabon20: "Take the top." CindyCan18: "Off?" Estabon20: "Then the short." CindyCan18: "Off? What about u? What are u waring?" Estabon20: "T shirt. Jean." CindyCan18: "Oh, can you tell me what to do now?" Estabon20: "No, you got to tell me what to do now?" CindyCan18: "Take off your pants and shorts." Estabon20: "I waring nice bikini shorts." CindyCan18: "Nice." Estabon20: "I take them off now and go to bed, OK."

Estabon20 signs off rather climactically. Eric speculates that maybe Estabon20 has gotten his jollies before splitting. Deciding to venture into the twentysomething chat room, Eric assumes yet another of his aliases, Huxley902. "I kinda lonely. Want to talk to someone," he types. Within seconds, Huxley902 gets a response from White615: "Hi. What are you up to tonight?" Huxley902: "I guess it really depends on what gender you are?" White615: "Tell me about yourself." Huxley902: "I'm 19, a guy actually. I like to play squash and read. I'm sort of an introvert. I like to listen to music and cook. You?" White615: "I'm 24, a gal actually. I love to read and listen to music." Huxley902: "Well, you're a gal. That's a start, eh? What music do you like?" White615: "You name it. I love it." Huxley902: "Dave Matthews Band?" White615: "Some." Huxley902: "What books? By the way, this is not the Grand Inquisition. Just wondering, that's all. Where do you live?" White615: "Sidney Sheldon. Arkansas." Huxley902: "You mean the mystery writer?" White615: "You like him?" Huxley902: "Never read him." White615: "He writes great, grisly thrillers." Huxley902: "Ewww. You are a most gruesome girl." White615: "He is actually a most challenging writer. I am, I mean I used to be an Emergency Medical Tech." Huxley902: "I am a literature student in Vancouver."

Eric pauses to pour himself another glass of wine. "Imagine. There are twenty-three million people out there doing this right now. How sick are we?" Eric doesn't answer his own question. Instead, he metamorphoses into the lovestruck but scholarly Huxley902 again.

White615: "I am fascinated by literature. Who are your favorite authors? What do you want to do when you graduate?" Huxley902: "Dostoyevsky. Roland Barthes. I want to be a professor when I graduate. By the way, you are not even mentioning sex at all." White615: "That is a great goal, to be a professor." Huxley902: "You are not offended by me mentioning sex, are you?" White615: "Oh no. I love honesty. What about Shakespeare?" Huxley902: "Shakespeare is good, but Canadian literature is great." White615: "I'm afraid I don't know very much about Canadian literature." Huxley902: "Really. But don't feel too bad. Nobody does. Just me. That's why I'm lonely." White615: "Then you will be a very famous professor of Canadian literature."

Eric downs his glass of wine and admits to being a little mystified: "What's happening? It seems that some people only want to chat in the chat room tonight. What a concept." Back to the keyboard. Huxley902: "Do you often get hassled by guys online? You are so very sweet." Eric reveals that this is a watershed question. White615, he thinks, is now deciding whether she'll reveal her true intentions.

Having pondered the question, White615 shoots back this response: "Not into sex." Ever the smoothie, Huxley902 offers consolation: "Know what you mean. So many perverts out there." White615: "You are right. People are so shallow." Huxley902: "You are so right, White. Thanks for sharing that. By the way, what's your real name? My real name is Eric and I'm most pleased to meet you."

Meanwhile, someone called Dude cuts into the conversation and offers Huxley902 a deal on some racy porno flicks: "Don't say i never done anything for you, dude." And then another missive lands. Marlon sends out an urgent plea: "i really want to talk to someone with shaved balls. i have issues, ok?"

We hear ya, Marlon. However, White615 decides to come clean with Huxley902: "My name is Cheryl. I come from Anderson." Huxley902: "Big town?" White615: "Ya gotta be joking. I was in a graduating class of 15." To demonstrate his sensitivity, Huxley902 dives into his Internet encyclopedia on the other part of the screen and searches for info about Anderson. He uncovers the Buford Manor Inn and Orville's Gourmet House. Huxley902 resumes his romance: "Ever heard of the Buford or Orville's?" White615: "No. This is a very small town, though. But that's very kind of you to ask." Huxley902: "I'm going to add you to my buddy list and we can have more great chats." White615: "Nite." Huxley902: "Gosh, you're sweet." White615: "Oh, you're such a charmer." Huxley902: "What do you look like?" White615: "I hope this doesn't turn you off. But my eyes get dark when I'm sassy." Energized now, Huxley902 fires back: "Sassy?"

Eric says White615 is a longterm project. But he sees possibilities. "Patience. It's all about patience. Huxley902 will demonstrate a maturity beyond his years and will eventually get to know White615 more intimately." For now, though, Eric, who has switched to swilling single-malt scotch, wants to play some more. He takes on one of his more precocious Internet identities, Lady Latonia, and enters a chat room for the thirtysomething contingent.

Lady Latonia: "Hello. I'm a classy lady from Montreal. I speak a bit of French and a bit of English and a bit of Spanish." To Lady Latonia's astonishment, this chat room appears to be inhabited exclusively by women. Lady Latonia: "What's going on here? Is this a lesbian room?" She is contacted immediately by Tooting Brain: "I can direct you to one if you wish . . ." Says Eric, "Is this sick or what? I'm a forty-eight-year-old father of two and I'm playing a lesbian." Nonetheless, he remains undeterred.

Tooting Brain: "Are you looking for lesbian support? I can help. I can be your friend." Lady Latonia: "Now that you mention it, I would prefer a lady in her early 20s, a kinky one too, who wants to do cyber online. In fact, I wish I could play with you, because you sound real nice and sensitive and seem to be quite understanding." Tooting Brain: "I already have a wife, if you catch my meaning." Lady Latonia: "So?" Tooting Brain: "Just go to the lesbian chat room, and maybe your prayers will be answered." Lady Latonia: "You're most kind." Tooting Brain: "Happy hunting."

Lady Latonia enters the specified lesbian chat room and immediately sends out her coordinates. Tricia the Ride Drifter is first to respond. Lady Latonia: "I'm 5' 8", shapely and I'm lookin for love." Tricia the Ride Drifter: "I'm 5' 2", 120 pounds and 36–D. I am also a passionate woman. But I need to know what I am talking to." Lady Latonia: "You mean 'who' you are talking to. Good grammar is very important to me." Tricia the Ride Drifter: "Yes, sorry."

Someone called Jake sends Lady Latonia salutations. Lady Latonia: "What are you doing here? This is a lesbian chat room. You should be ashamed of yourself. Go away."

Back to the Ride Drifter. Lady Latonia: "Language really turns me on." Tricia the Ride Drifter: "Me too. In fact, I am known for my grammer skills. However I have been drinken tonight." Lady Latonia: "This turns me on." Tricia the Ride Drifter: "How much?"

On line 2, Jake won't relent: "I'm back." Lady Latonia: "You're a fucking guy, aren't you?" Jake: "No." Lady Latonia: "Yes, you are." Jake: "I have a confession. I'm a guy." Lady Latonia: "Really." Jake: "I'm here looking for my girlfriend. She has left me for another woman. Are you her?" Lady Latonia: "I don't think so. Are you a jerk?" Jake: "Maybe. Bye now."

On line 1, Tricia the Ride Drifter is sending photos to Lady Latonia: "This is me with my girlfriend Mocha. This is me with my boyfriend Billy. And this is just me." If these images truly are of Tricia the Ride Drifter, then Lady Latonia has hit the motherlode. Lady Latonia, wise beyond her years, figures they are stock shots that Tricia the Ride Drifter has captured from a Web site for models. No matter. Lady Latonia: "Wow, you're beautiful. Give me your tongue right now and I'll make it dance." Tricia the Ride Drifter: "I would love to make love to you. Oh, Canada. Candoooo, Canada. Oh my gowwwwwd. I love to lick." Lady Latonia: "Do it to me! Do it now! I want you real badly!" Tricia the Ride Drifter: "You will have to call me for me to believe your a female. I'm getting strange vibes. This is BOGUSSS."

Eric is amused. "I'm sensing some tension here. She's getting hostile." Tricia the Ride Drifter: "Please call immediately. Here is my phone number. I think I'm ready to love you. But first I must know if your really a female person." Lady Latonia tries to turn the tables: "You're a fucking guy, aren't you?" Tricia the Ride Drifter: "No way. You are." Lady Latonia: "Admit it. You're a guy." Tricia the Ride Drifter: "Prove it." Lady Latonia: "I don't think there is enough honesty in this relationship. Nite." Tricia the Ride Drifter: "Nite." On line 3, Hellfire is offering to send pictures of his lesbian sister to all interested parties. With a brother like that . . . It's been almost four hours since Eric first signed on. "It's interesting to play with people's perversions, but like anything else, it gets incredibly boring after a while. Maybe, if I were really a single, lonely lady, I'd take this a little more seriously." Eric guesses that some people really do use the Net to find real partners. "But ninety percent are real sickos, just like me." He grins. "You just can't believe anyone. It's all a masquerade. The idea is to convince the other party that you are who you're pretending to be. One time, I asked a guy to go down on me. He said okay. Then I told him it was my period. He immediately signed off. But I convinced him, right?"

With that revelation, Eric concedes that it's a distinct possibility everyone in the lesbian chat room this evening was a guy. "That's so typical of men." I believe this is Lady Latonia talking.

Margo comes in to bid us good night. "It's all about role-playing, honey," he tells her, sounding somewhat disenchanted. "No one is who they pretend to be." Counters the no-nonsense Margo, "Of course not, dear. If any of these people were who they say they are, they wouldn't be online. They'd have lives."

Amen.

EPILOGUE

The money and the power and the fantasy notwithstanding, it all comes down to survival. Sex, that is. I am passing on this stunning factoid to the busboy I encountered six months earlier. I am back at the Japanese restaurant where my odyssey began after I'd been successfully plied with way too much saki by my sage publisher.

To prove my thesis to the earnest busboy, I relay a story about Chinese scientists in Beijing. At their wits' end, these noble men of science were hoping to spur the sex drive of giant pandas by showing them porn videos. "As part of the pandas' education, we make those that are sexually inept watch videos of other pandas having sex," explained Zhang Hemin, director of the China Giant Panda Research and Conservation Center in the southwestern province of Sichuan. Evidently, the center, which is home to forty-six pandas, a third of the world's entire population of pandas in captivity, had enjoyed some success with its sex education program.

This program also entailed arranging for young pandas to watch their elders mate, as they would in the wild. Before entering the program, eighty percent of the center's males were impotent. This figure has now fallen to sixty percent. The center is also allowing male and female pandas to socialize and play together rather than spending all their time cooped up alone. But Zhang dismissed recent media reports that his center planned to feed its male pandas Viagra. The reports apparently derived from a Chinese journalist who had misunderstood a joke, officials at the center insisted. However, in 1992, the center did experiment with traditional herbal aphrodisiacs. Sadly, the drugs merely made the males aggressive with their mates.

There are an estimated one thousand giant pandas left in the wild, all of them in China. But if the blue movies take, I tell the busboy, the panda will no longer be an endangered species. "Great news, right?" The busboy seems disappointed. Slowly shaking his head, he says, "This is what you've learned after six months in the sex capitals of the world? Panda porn! Where's the dirt? Don't hold back, grasshopper — tell me what you really discovered."

Well, if you insist. I discovered that my love for NFL football was greater than I had ever imagined — so much so that I willingly left a roomful of naked, well-endowed porno stars in Las Vegas to catch playoff action on the tube in my room. I discovered that the one thing porn stars covet more than money is . . . wait for it . . . romance. And with just one mate . . . Sheesh. I also discovered that some dominatrixes would prefer to walk their dogs on a leash for free than walk their clients on a choker for a pile of cash. And that some find a visit to a hardcore Dutch sex museum about as titillating as a visit to the local butcher shop. And that many Frenchmen find women sexier clothed than they are naked. And that many swingers have more moral scruples than most straight folk I know. And that there are few more ridiculous spectacles than middle-aged male lawyers strutting in lederhosen on fetish nights. And that some women love filthy jokes more than their fellas do. And that some men would prefer to bite down on burgers rather than surgically enhanced lap dancers. And that Internet chat rooms could signal the end of Western Civilization as we know it.

"Anything else?" the busboy asks with a tone of great dejection. "Yes, as a matter of fact," I counter. "I'll never be able to look at a banana again without blushing and/or getting queasy."

The busboy persists: "But would you do it all over again if you could?" "In an Amsterdam moment," I reply. He smiles. "But," I add, "not necessarily in the next one — moment, that is." He sighs.

The busboy wants to say something, but words fail him at this point. Fortunately, a man sitting alone at a nearby table has no such problem. This elegant-looking gentleman, sporting an ascot and an impressive handlebar mustache, feels compelled to say: "I couldn't help but overhear your conversation and if you don't mind my saying, I do believe I have the solution. I can save civilization."

"So speak!" the busboy and I cry in unison. "My newest invention is the Universal Sex Wheel," begins the gent. Just when I thought I had seen and heard everything. Universal Sex Wheel? The mind boggles. I ask whether it's some kind of kinky Ferris wheel. Or multicultural torture device. "Not quite," he states. He's playing his cards close to his vest, but upon further prodding, he does reveal that the Universal Sex Wheel can determine the periods of the year when a couple will be most sexually in sync and in heat.

The busboy and I are both speechless. The gentleman is not. His name is David Greenacre. Turns out that he is an inventor — dice and board-games and wheel-of-fortune division. He is listed in *The International Who's Who of Intellectuals*. What all of this really means is that Greenacre must, sadly, toil as a painter and plasterer and a doorman to pay the rent until he strikes it rich with one of his inventions, or until mankind decides to cut its genius inventors a subsistence wage. Yet Greenacre is undaunted.

Born in Caracas, Venezuela, raised in the Bahamas, and educated in England, David Greenacre had initially hoped to follow in the footsteps of his father — a member of the Order of the British Empire — and become a CEO. This didn't pan out, but he still boldly predicts that the Universal Sex Wheel will be his ticket to the top. While he is circumspect about his methodology, he indicates that there is a secret, heretofore unknown, mathematical formula underlying most, if not all, human behavior. He refuses to reveal this secret formula just yet. But lest you get the impression that Greenacre lacks an earthly focus, be assured that he is a true humanitarian: "It would be fantastic to be able to make people aware that the reality of happiness and heartbreak is mathematically based and, hence, completely unavoidable." And Greenacre is also as entrepreneurial as the Hef himself. "My ultimate fantasy? Simple. Selling one of these wheels to Oprah and then appearing on her show." Duh.

The sex carnival moves on.